TI

A Woman's Guide To

A WOMAN'S GUIDE TO BREAST HEALTH

CATH CIRKET
Consultant editor: Penny Mares
Published in conjunction with the
NATIONAL EXTENSION COLLEGE

Foreword by Jinty Blanckenhagen,
Director of the Breast Care and Mastectomy Association

GRAPEVINE

First edition 1989

© National Extension College
Illustrations by Jane Bottomley
Cartoons by Angela Martin

British Library Cataloguing in Publication Data

Cirket, Cath
  Breast health
  1. Women. Breasts. Diseases
  I. Title
  618.1'9

ISBN 0 7225 1790 4

Grapevine is an imprint of Thorsons Publishers Limited, Wellingborough, Northamptonshire NN8 2RQ, England.

Printed in Great Britain by Biddles Limited, Guildford, Surrey
Typeset by MJL Limited, Hitchin, Hertfordshire

10 9 8 7 6 5 4 3 2 1

Contents

Foreword

by Jinty Blanckenhagen
Director of the Breast Care
and Mastectomy of Great Britain

The author of this well researched and useful book not only provides women with a comprehensive range of information and sources for further knowledge, but also conveys to the reader a sense of personal involvement in each topic. Recognizing that each individual brings her own feelings and experiences to the normal happy events and the difficult crises in our lives, she has stressed the ability in us to learn, adapt and cope in our own unique way with the enjoyment of good health and the problems of poor health.

The scope of the book covers the current issues surrounding treatments available today in Britain for benign breast disease and breast cancer. There are suggestions about issues women may wish to think about and discuss together, along with questions to ask those who may be able to provide the answers. Hopefully women reading this book will feel more confident about being involved in some of the decisions affecting their lives.

Jinty Blanckenhagen
Director
BREAST CARE AND MASTECTOMY ASSOCIATION OF GREAT BRITAIN

About this book

This is a book about breast problems and breast disease. It is for all women, but especially for women who are feeling anxious about their breasts or who are facing a worrying diagnosis or treatment. Because women will want different kinds of information at different times in their lives, the book has been written as a handbook so that women can dip into it when they need to.

The book argues for a whole-person (or holistic) approach to breast problems and breast disease. It looks at traditional and complementary treatments as well as those offered by modern medicine and discusses ways in which we can help ourselves to better health. The book aims to enable women to make informed choices about how they are treated. Most women find it difficult to assert themselves when faced with a formal situation in a surgery or hospital. Practical suggestions are made, therefore, in several chapters to overcome these problems so that women can find the confidence to voice their worries and make any decisions they need to.

Throughout the text most health professionals are referred to as 'she'. This avoids the awkwardness of s/he (or him/her) and any stereotyping of doctors and surgeons being exclusively male and nursing and other support workers being female. The exception to this is hospital consultants, as few women will have the opportunity of seeing a woman consultant. Many women would prefer to be treated by a woman consultant or doctor if they were to discover breast disease. Hopefully it won't be too long before this is a reality.

At the end of each chapter a short reading list is suggested for those women who wish to read more. (Where possible paperbacks have been recommended.) Ideally these should be available in any library or health clinic. If this is not the case where you live, use the list to request that these books are stocked so that they are available to you and other women in your area.

Most women are deeply afraid of cancer and find it very difficult to read about breast cancer without becoming extremely anxious. By looking at *all* breast problems and diseases, this book hopes to minimize undue anxiety. It is important that the mystery and fear surrounding cancer doesn't prevent us from being properly informed and able to act in our own best interests. It's also important that women who have breast cancer have support and solidarity in living with this serious disease.

The book is primarily for women but it is also designed to be shared and discussed with partners and friends. It could be used as the basis for a course on breast health. Hopefully the experiences in it will generate discussions and humour, both of which have played an important part in writing the book and in the lives of the many women who have contributed to it.

Acknowledgements

The following people have contributed ideas and criticisms in the writing of this book. Some are health professionals and others are women in different situations and backgrounds. I would like to thank them for their contributions which have been extremely helpful. They are: Nicki Bennet, Julie Berry, Anne Birch, Naomi Brent, Moya Burns, Jennifer Caseldine, Angela Cirket, Stella Cirket, Theresa Cirket, Cath Clarke, Elizabeth Cosgrave, Jane Dorner, Linda Ellis, Judy Farrel, Peter Fenton, Leslie Ferguson, Jenny Fortune, Fi Frances, Janet Gagehan, Katy Gardner, Linda Grant, Shirley Hetherington, Angela Holt, Rachel Hope, Helen Ives, Russell Keeley, Mavis Kirkham, Em Lawless, Liz Lawrence, Marina Lewycka, Avril Lyons, Penny Mares, Anne Meehan, Anthony Meehan, Michael Meehan, Ros Morpeth, Annie Neligan, Maggie Norton, Brenda O'Brian, Mary Ann Orme, Anne Parker, Rosemary Pratt, Kate Richards, Jenny River, Mena Sarin, Margaret Shand, Mary Shand, Dudley Sinnett, Carol Smith, Ann Staniland, Adele Stanley, Donal Stevens, Mary Stoddard, Hilary Templar, Freda Thompson, Laura Tolley, Vicky Tongsri, Mary Twomey, Julia Unwin, Kate Vickers, Cesar Viracca, Bisi Williams, Maureen Williams, Catherine Wills, Diana Woodward. I would also like to thank the staff of the Breast Care and Mastectomy Association, Cancerlink, Bacup, The British Holistic Medical Association, The Bristol Cancer Help Centre and New Approaches to Cancer.

I would particularly like to thank Vera Beining, Chris Gifford, Cynthia James, Gwyn Lauteburg, Peggy Moore, Barbara Rosenblum, Margaret Selmes, Jo Spence and Wendy Wells. The book is dedicated to them and to the many thousands of women who are living with breast disease.

While acknowledging the contribution made by those above, any weaknesses in the text are mine alone.   Cath Cirket.

CHAPTER ONE

Our breasts and how we feel about them

This chapter describes different women's experience and feelings about their breasts. It looks at some of the wider issues concerning our bodies and our sexuality and stresses the importance of a whole-person approach to our health.

Our breasts are glands which produce milk to feed our young, a function we have in common with all mammals. The term 'mammal' comes from mammae or mammary glands which are the technical names for breasts. In our society, women's breasts have an importance attached to them far beyond this ability to feed our children. Our breasts are regarded as a symbol of womanhood and of sexual arousal. How society sees us may well be different from how we see ourselves but few women are able to free themselves completely from the models of 'beauty' and 'attractiveness', handed to us by the media or learnt in other ways.

Breast development

From early adolescence, we are conscious of the changes taking place in our bodies and this is most visible in the development of our breasts. Many women remember this time with a mixture of pride, amusement, excitement and pain.

> There was one girl at school who was very shapely and grown-up while I was flat-chested and felt inadequate. We were having a shower one day and, to my surprise, I discovered this girl was just as flat-chested as me only she used to stuff her bra with nylons!

As girls we may have worried that our breasts developed more slowly or more quickly than other girls' breasts.

> They used to call me 'drainpipe' when I was at school because I was so flat-chested.

Young women can be extremely sensitive about the development of their breasts. Careless comments or a lack of openness about the changes taking place can lead to many heartaches.

> When I was sixteen, this boy I was going out with said to me 'Your looks are all right but your tits are rubbish.' I was terribly hurt.

The effects of teasing or embarrassment about our breasts sometimes remain with us in adult life. 'Round' shoulders, hugging ourselves or folding our arms at every opportunity are often echoes of an earlier need to protect ourselves and our breasts from public view.

Breast size and shape

Whatever our breast size, we have the milk-producing capacity which allows us to breastfeed children should we want to do so. How we feel about the size of our breasts varies from woman to woman and has a lot to do with how we feel about our bodies in general.

> I only began to feel good about my breasts when I became pregnant and while I was breastfeeding. My breasts were larger and somehow more a part of me. The whole experience has made me feel better about them.

A number of women have lopsided breasts where one breast is lower than the other and some women have one breast larger than the other. This is nothing to worry about. If your breasts become lopsided or unbalanced in the space of a few months, then it is worth checking to make sure nothing is wrong.

Other women may have an inverted nipple in one or both breasts. (An inverted nipple turns inwards rather than stands erect). Many women worry that they won't be able to breastfeed with an inverted nipple but this is rarely the case.

Sexual feelings

When we are sexually aroused changes take place in our breasts. They become enlarged and more sensitive. The nipples stand erect.

Some women notice these changes and others don't. Having our breasts caressed can be an important part of lovemaking in the sensations we feel and in our enjoyment of sex.

Mothers who decide to breastfeed will discover a range of sensations in their breasts — both painful and pleasurable — and some women find breastfeeding intensely pleasurable and arousing.

> I decided to breastfeed because I thought it would be better for the baby. Nobody told me how much pleasure I would get from it.

Other women may feel torn between enjoying breastfeeding their child and enjoying their breasts in lovemaking.

> My breasts are very important to me sexually. I was really pleased to stop breastfeeding so that I could have my breasts to myself again, if you know what I mean.

Our breasts may also be sexually arousing for our partners, and they are certainly a source of comfort and enjoyment in the many hugs we have with friends, relatives and particularly children.

Images of women in our society

Our breasts are important to us as women. They are a positive part of our womanhood. At the same time, society's ideas of women can make us feel that our breasts restrict and stereotype us.

Wherever we look around us, in newspapers, magazines, films, advertisements, we see images of women's breasts. The Page Three image of firm rounded breasts with upturned nipples is difficult to live up to and sometimes makes us feel inadequate and unattractive. Fashions change and the ideal size and shape of women's bodies change with them. No wonder our feelings about our breasts are contradictory.

In our society women's breasts are an important symbol of sexual attraction to men. How we look can become more important than who we are. Comments in the street may appear to flatter but they can also be unwanted and make us feel undervalued as human beings.

> I have to be careful what I wear. If I wear something too tight or too revealing men stare at me in the street. Sometimes they make remarks. I suppose I should be flattered, but I just feel embarrassed.

For many women their self-confidence and sense of self-esteem is closely linked to how they look and whether they are visually attractive to their partners and to the world at large. We are taught by every advert and Page Three pin-up that appearances count. Because of these pressures many women have mixed feelings about their bodies.

> I feel as if I'm two people: my mind and my personality, which are the real *me* and my body which I feel alienated from. I find it very difficult to look at myself in the mirror and say 'Don't you look nice?' Instead I say 'Never mind, you're a nice person and that's what counts.'

Standing up to the stereotypes

Talking to other women can help us to feel better about our bodies and to resist society's pressures about who's attractive and who isn't.

> I started going to a group for women with eating problems about a year ago. So many women have eating problems and it makes no difference if they're fat or thin. I never realized that. It's made me feel a lot more confident about myself and my body.

Voicing our feelings about ourselves and knowing that we're not the only ones with doubts or problems is an important way of gaining confidence. Learning to feel good about our bodies and our breasts may need the help and support of a women's group or a well-woman clinic and some women will need to go to a counsellor or therapist. Together women can work out ways of challenging the hurtful comments, jokes and silences which may help to undermine us. We can also try to educate those close to us to be sensitive to our feelings about our bodies, our breasts and our sexual needs.

Your local library will have a list of women's groups or a contact number to find out about these. Your doctor should be able to help you find a well-woman clinic or a counsellor or therapist. Your local education authority can tell you about women's health classes, yoga and other adult education classes which might be helpful. There may also be local campaigns about sexual harassment at work, equal opportunities for women and other issues that affect our health and our lives.

Further reading

Angela Phillips and Jill Rakusen (eds), *Our Bodies — Our Selves*, (Penguin Books, 1987) is a very useful reference book on women's health.

Suzie Orbach, *Fat is a Feminist Issue* (Arrow Books, 1988) looks at the problematic relationship between women and food.

CHAPTER TWO
How our breasts work

Understanding how our breasts work helps us to understand the causes and treatment of breast disease. This chapter looks at the structure of the breast and at different types of breast tissue: the milk-producing system, the cells which shape the breast, the blood supply and the lymphatic system. It also looks at the way

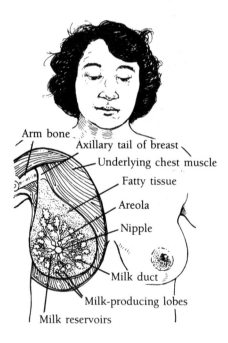

Figure 1 Front view of the breast.

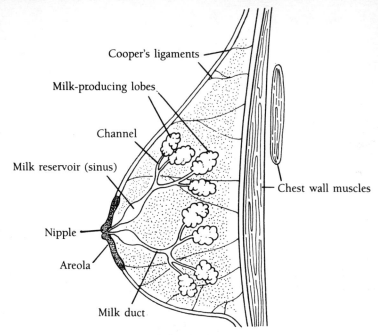

Cooper's ligaments

Milk-producing lobes

Channel

Milk reservoir (sinus)

Nipple

Areola

Milk duct

Chest wall muscles

Figure 2 Side view of the breast. (Adapted from Breast Cancer: the facts *by Michael Baum, 1981, 1988 © Michael Baum, published by Oxford University Press.)*

hormones influence breast tissue and outlines the changes which take place during our reproductive lives.

The milk-producing system

Each breast is a milk-producing (mammary) gland containing 16 — 20 milk-producing lobes, which spread out in a rough circle from a centre point behind the nipple, and up towards the armpit (axilla). Each lobe is made up of many lobules, which collect milk from hundreds of milk-producing cells. From the lobes, the milk is transferred down channels (ducts). These widen out into small saclike reservoirs (sinuses), which are connected to the nipple.

Most women find that their nipples are very sensitive to touch or changes in temperature. This is because each nipple contains many small muscle fibres which contract when stimulated, causing the nipple to stand erect. Around the nipple is a darker area called the areola which contains very small glands, which may expand during pregnancy, boosting the milk supply.

The shape of the breast

Our breasts also contain fat and fibrous tissue which help contribute to their size and shape. Fibrous tissue helps to give the breast firmness and support, particularly the fibrous ligaments known as 'Cooper's ligaments' which support the breasts against the underlying chest muscle. As we grow older our breasts tend to lose this firmness as these ligaments lose elasticity.

The blood supply

The blood supply carries nourishment and oxygen to every part of the body, including the breasts, through a network of blood vessels. The larger blood vessels (arteries) carry oxygen-rich blood from the heart to body tissue. These branch into smaller and smaller vessels — the smallest are called capillaries. Veins carry away the oxygen-depleted blood back to the heart.

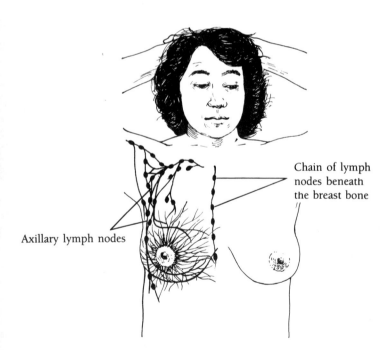

Chain of lymph nodes beneath the breast bone

Axillary lymph nodes

Figure 3 The lymphatic system in the area of the breast (Adapted from Breast Cancer *by J. Davey, BUPA, 1974.)*

The lymphatic system

Equally important to the health of body tissue is the lymphatic system which forms an important part of the immune system. Lymphatic channels clear away many unwanted products from body tissue. In the breast, these channels drain outwards from the breast towards the axillary (armpit) lymph nodes, the shoulder lymph nodes and the nodes beneath the breast bone.

How hormones work

Hormones are natural chemical signals produced by a number of glands in the body. (A gland is any tissue which produces specialized body substances.) Hormone signals circulate throughout the body, telling cells how to behave. Each body cell is 'bathed' with many different hormones all the time. Some hormones act directly on cells and some trigger other hormones into action (see checklist on page 20). In the course of a woman's life, her breasts will go through a number of natural changes, and many of these are controlled by the activity of hormones.

Starting periods (puberty)

A young girl's breasts begin to develop at puberty, around the same time that her periods start. The hormones oestrogen and progesterone play an important part in telling the body when periods should start and in regulating the monthly cycle.

Monthly cycle

During the course of the monthly cycle, many women are aware of changes in their breasts. At ovulation, the time when the egg is produced — roughly a fortnight before your next period — your breasts may feel more sensitive. Towards the end of the cycle your breasts may well feel lumpy or swollen. This is due to the influence of oestrogen and progesterone as they prepare the body for the possibility of pregnancy. If the egg is not fertilized, hormone levels fall and your breasts return to their normal size soon after the start of your period.

Pregnancy

When a woman becomes pregnant, the egg is fertilized shortly after ovulation and the production of oestrogen and progesterone continues and increases. The breasts then become noticeably larger and this is one of the earliest signs of pregnancy.

A number of hormones are released during pregnancy and play an important part in preparing the breasts for milk production. (see 'Checklist of hormones which affect our breasts' on page 20).

Breastfeeding

The first time a baby feeds it receives not milk but a rich yellowish substance called colostrum. This prepares the baby's gut for digesting milk. It also passes on to the baby some of the mother's immunity to illness. After a number of feeds the breasts become very full of milk. They may feel painful and lumpy and small amounts of milk may leak from the nipples but this settles down as feeding is established.

Change of life (menopause)

As women reach the end of their child-bearing years, the ovaries stop the production of a monthly egg and the production of oestrogen and progesterone falls. Glandular breast tissue begins to be replaced by fat cells.

Many of the symptoms of the change of life — hot flushes, irregular bleeding and dryness in the vagina — are caused by these hormonal changes. Many women have been able to adjust to these changes without serious distress, but some women, experiencing severe symptoms, can be helped by Hormone Replacement Therapy (HRT) for long or short periods (see page 44 for further comments on HRT).

Checklist of hormones which affect our breasts

Hormone	Where it is produced	What it does
Growth hormone	The pituitary gland	Stimulates and controls growth throughout the body
Oestrogen	The ovaries (main source), the adrenal cortex (in small quantities), the placenta; fat cells and cells of the	Together with growth hormone, is responsible for the development of milk ducts in the breast; causes changes in

	large bowel also produce oestrogen	the ducts and lobules during the monthly cycle and during pregnancy
Progesterone	The ovaries (main source), and the placenta	Together with growth hormone, is responsible for the development of the milk-producing lobules; causes changes in the ducts and lobules during the monthly cycle and during pregnancy
Luteinizing hormone and follicle stimulating hormone	The pituitary gland	Triggers and controls the development and release of eggs from the ovaries; triggers and controls the production of oestrogen and progesterone
Human chorionic gonadotrophin	The placenta	Halts normal monthly cycle during pregnancy; suppresses prolactin (milk-producing hormone) until after birth
Prolactin	The pituitary gland	Responsible, with progesterone, for the development of the milk-producing lobules; responsible for milk production, once oestrogen and progesterone have prepared the way

Oxytocin	The pituitary gland	Stimulates labour at the end of pregnancy; stimulates milk flow as the baby sucks

During our reproductive lives, our breasts undergo many changes. Understanding these changes is important if we want to know how our breasts work. It is also useful for us to know what lies where. Armed with this knowledge, we are in a better position to understand what is happening if we discover a problem in our breasts.

Further reading

Michael Baum, *Breast Cancer: The Facts* (Oxford University Press, 1988), gives a clear explanation of the structure and function of the breast with useful diagrams (see Chapter 3).

Patrick Holford, *The Whole Health Manual* (Thorsons, 1985), gives a useful explanation of how the body works which is easy to read (see Chapter 1).

Angela Phillips and Jill Rakusen, *Our Bodies—Our Selves* (Penguin Books, 1987), looks at all aspects of women's health and has a useful section on periods, pregnancy and the menopause.

The Biology of Health and Disease, Book IV, produced by the Open University, gives a technical but thorough explanation of the body's systems.

CHAPTER THREE

Breast problems and diseases of the breast

Many women will have a breast problem at some point in their lives. Most of these will be linked to hormonal changes in the body, some will produce unpleasant symptoms and some will pose the possibility of a serious disease. If you are reading this section because you have a breast problem, bear in mind that the great majority of breast problems and breast diseases are not cancer.

This chapter looks at some common breast problems, non-cancerous breast conditions and some of the different cancers of the breast. A checklist of symptoms and diseases is set out at the end. (Information about treatments for these problems and diseases is given in Chapters 11—17.)

If you are worried...

Reading about the symptoms of breast disease makes some women anxious. It is worth bearing in mind that your breasts undergo many changes in your life, particularly during your reproductive years, and that these are normal and no cause for concern.

If you discover a change in your breasts, particularly if you discover a lump, you may well feel very anxious because of the fear of cancer. By informing yourself about different diseases of the breast, you can begin to consider what may be wrong. But if you are worried, you should seek help. It will take the expertise of doctors and other health professionals to make a proper diagnosis should something be wrong.

Breast problems

Problems relating to the monthly cycle

Pain You may get breast pain (mastalgia) at any time of the month but it is usually most noticeable leading up to a period. It may be localized pain or a general feeling of soreness and tenderness and can be severe at times. Some women experience pain under their arms where glandular tissue reaches up into the armpit.

Swelling Some women experience a tight, bloated sensation in their breasts leading up to a period. Others experience lumpiness or thickening. This swelling is due to increased glandular activity and increased fluid in the breast. Once your period starts this bloated feeling usually goes.

Leaking nipples Sometimes a woman who is not pregnant or breastfeeding may find that her nipples leak drops of milk. This can happen as a result of taking the Pill or other tablets which stimulate the production of prolactin. Once the hormonal balance is restored, the leaking usually stops. If leaking nipples persist, this can be due to overproduction of prolactin from the pituitary gland. This should be checked out by a simple blood test to make sure there is no underlying disorder.

Problems in pregnancy and breastfeeding
Accessory nipples Accessory or secondary nipples are small additional nipples usually found in front of the armpit or below the breasts. They are nothing to worry about and often go unnoticed though they may become tender and swollen when breastfeeding begins and leak drops of milk. This will settle down once breastfeeding (or bottle-feeding) is established.

Leaking nipples during pregnancy During pregnancy some women find that their nipples leak drops of milk or blood. This is nothing to worry about and settles down once breastfeeding begins.

Inverted nipples and breastfeeding An inverted nipple turns inwards rather than stands erect when it is stimulated. Some women who have inverted nipples (one or both breasts) may have a problem encouraging the nipple to stand out. Only very rarely are women unable to breastfeed because of inverted nipples (see page 12).

Sore and cracked nipples Sore or cracked nipples can occur in breastfeeding. This sometimes happens if the baby is not sucking properly. Soaps and detergents can dry up the natural oils in the area of the nipples causing soreness. Eczema, a skin rash, can lead to dry, cracked nipples. (Eczema can easily spread from another part of the body.)

Mastitis Mastitis is an infection in the milk ducts which may develop in the later stages of pregnancy or when breastfeeding. The breast feels sore and inflamed and you may feel feverish. There may also be a discharge of pus from the nipple. The lymph nodes in the armpit sometimes become enlarged as a result of infection.

Mastitis can sometimes become a chronic infection. It is thought that this can be due to overuse of antibiotics in treating the infection. Stopping the antibiotics can sometimes cure the complaint. An unusual form of mastitis, which does not occur during pregnancy and breastfeeding, is not due to infection. It is caused by chemical changes in the duct tissue which create similar inflammatory symptoms. This condition is called 'plasma cell mastitis' or 'periductal mastitis'.

The term 'mastitis' is often used by doctors to describe *any* painful breast condition. If you don't have a breast infection or inflammation and are told you have mastitis, you might want to ask your doctor for more information.

Breast abscesses If a breast infection goes untreated, a breast abscess can develop in one of the milk ducts causing localized pain and swelling. If it is near the surface, it will look like a boil. You may also feel feverish.

(See Chapter 6 for details of breast care in pregnancy and breastfeeding.)

Non-cancerous diseases of the breast

Some non-cancerous breast conditions are brought about by imbalances in oestrogen and progesterone levels and inappropriate new cell growth in the breast. This may result in a lump or lumpiness, pain, tenderness, nipple discharge, inverted nipples or any combination of these. Here is a list of the most common breast complaints. Remember, the majority of breast problems and diseases are *not* cancer.

Cysts A breast cyst is a balloon-like capsule filled with fluid which forms in a duct or lobule. Most cysts are small and form in clusters. Some are larger and can be felt as a smooth, rounded lump in the breast which moves easily under the skin. Some cysts grow slowly while others appear quite suddenly. Sometimes if the lining of a cyst is broken, it can dissolve and disappear with no further problem.

A cyst may form in any part of the breast where there is duct

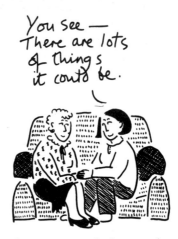

or lobe tissue but the most usual place is the upper outer part of the breast. A woman can have several cysts at one time and these may be in one or both breasts. They may be painful and tender to touch and they can also, occasionally, produce a nipple discharge. If a cyst grows very large, the shape of the breast can be distorted but this will go once the cyst is drained.

Cysts occur more frequently in childless women and are most likely to develop in women in their late thirties, forties and early fifties.

Fibroadenomas and lactational adenomas A fibroadenoma usually forms a well-defined firm lump which is easily felt. It also moves around freely under the skin surface. Fibroadenomas develop when there is increased cell growth in fibrous (fibro-) and glandular (-adeno) tissue. Sometimes several appear in one or both breasts, particularly in the upper outer part of the breast.

Fibroadenomas can develop during pregnancy. These tend to grow more rapidly and densely and are sometimes called lactational adenomas.

Younger women under the age of thirty are most likely to develop a fibroadenoma but women in their thirties and forties can also develop the condition.

Cystosarcoma phyllodes Cystosarcoma phyllodes is closely related to a fibroadenoma but tends to produce a harder lump which can sometimes grow quite large. Occasionally young girls develop this condition but it is most likely to occur in women in their thirties, forties and early fifties.

Fibrous disease Fibrous disease occurs when fibrous growth replaces glandular tissue. This new growth develops into a painless irregular lump which is easily felt and quite hard. Fibrous growths do not move around as easily as a cyst or fibroadenoma. They are mostly found in the upper outer portion of the breast and are more common between the ages of 35 and 55.

Fibroadenosis Fibroadenosis develops if there is a general increase in fibrous and glandular growth. This can produce areas of thickening and lumpiness in the breasts which can be painful and sore. It is most likely to occur in women in their forties and fifties.

Sclerosing adenosis When increased growth in glandular tissue becomes hardened and feels knobbly, the condition is called sclerosing adenosis (sclerosing means hardening). This condition tends to produce easily felt lumps and lumpiness as well as pain and tenderness. If a duct under the nipple is affected, this may cause the nipple to turn inwards.

Sclerosing adenosis usually affects women in their forties and fifties.

Fibrocystic disease Some doctors use the term fibrocystic disease to cover *any* non-cancerous cell growth in the ducts and lobules of the breast. This can include solitary cysts, fibroadenomas, fibrous growths, as well as fibroadenosis and sclerosing adenosis since all these conditions involve increased growth in the ducts and lobules of the breast. But fibrocystic disease is also the term used to describe clusters of small cysts which become surrounded by increased fibrous growth. It can cause considerable pain and tenderness and the breasts will feel lumpy. This is a common condition in women between 35 and 50.

Intraductal papillomas An intraductal papilloma is a small wartlike growth occurring in a large milk duct beneath the nipple. Some are too small to feel. If they are large enough, you will feel a pea-sized lump. A common symptom is a nipple discharge varying in colour from bloody to yellowish green. A nipple discharge is less likely if the intraductal papilloma grows in a duct away from the nipple.

Occasionally an intraductal papilloma can cause the nipple to turn inwards or cause dimpling in the surrounding skin. There may also be some inflammation but this is rare.

Intraductal papillomas are not usually painful although if a duct fills with fluid, you may have a feeling of uncomfortable fullness which is only relieved if the fluid is drained.

Duct ectasia Duct ectasia occurs when a duct enlarges and fills with cellular waste products producing a sticky multicoloured discharge and, sometimes, a burning or itching sensation in and around the nipples which can also be painful. The condition can affect many ducts in one or both breasts.

Gradually the diseased ducts become fibrous and hard, pulling the nipples inward, leaving a hard lumpy area beneath. Other symptoms of this fibrous process are dimpling in the skin or redness in the immediate area. The lymph nodes in the armpit may become enlarged.

Duct ectasia usually occurs in women in their forties and occasionally in older women. It is not a common condition.

Lipomas Like fibrous and glandular tissue, fat tissue can also develop new cell growth. These are called lipomas. They are painless, well-defined lumps, with no other symptoms. Lipomas occur frequently in other parts of the body and occasionally they develop in the breast.

Fat necrosis Fat necrosis means death of fat cells and this can occasionally happen as a result of injury, as part of the ageing process or if you lose weight very rapidly. The dead cells are replaced by fibrous tissue causing a hard, irregular lump. Other symptoms can include pain and tenderness, dimpling of the skin and enlarged lymph nodes in the armpit.

Cancers of the breast

The symptoms of breast cancer

All of the symptoms described here are often symptoms of noncancerous breast conditions and may have nothing to do with breast cancer. (See the full checklist of symptoms on page 31.)

Most breast cancers begin by developing a painless, hard lump often situated in the upper outer portion of the breast. If the cancer develops in the ducts beneath the nipple, there may be a discharge or the ducts may shrink, pulling the nipple inwards.

Sometimes a cancer can travel along the fibrous ligaments, pulling them inwards, causing the skin to dimple. If a cancer begins near the skin surface, there may be localized soreness, unusual thickening and possibly an open wound (ulceration). Skin which takes on the appearance of orange peel can also be a sign of an underlying cancer (the pitted texture indicates that many tiny ligament endings have been disturbed).

Pain and discomfort in the breast or in the armpit (or upper arm) is unusual but can't be ruled out as a symptom of cancer. Enlarged lymph nodes can also signal a cancer in the breast.

Different types of breast cancer

Breast cancers fall into two main types: those which stay within the ducts or lobules (non-invasive or *in situ* cancers) and those which spread into surrounding tissue in the breast and elsewhere (invasive cancers). In some cases, non-invasive cancers can become invasive, or both types can be present at the same time.

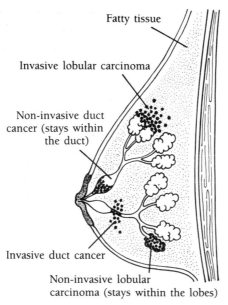

Figure 4 Invasive and non-invasive cancers (Adapted from Breast Cancer: the facts *by Michael Baum, published by Oxford University Press.)*

Non-invasive (in situ) cancers

Intraductal cancer Intraductal cancers (*intra* meaning within) occur in the milk ducts and usually develop into lumps which can be easily felt, particularly when the cancer occurs in one of the large ducts. The lump may feel irregular to touch and is usually painless.

Lobular carcinoma in situ These cancers occur in the lobules. They are often too small to feel and will only show up on a mammogram. They are usually painless.

Invasive cancers

Invasive duct cancer The majority of breast cancers (about 90 per cent) develop in the lining of the milk ducts. The most common cancer is called scirrhous cancer. This produces a hard, irregular lump (scirrhous means hard). Some cancers have a number of different cell types in them (see below).

Invasive lobular cancer About 8 per cent of breast cancers will begin in the lobules. These may develop into a lump or they may simply produce an area of localized thickening.

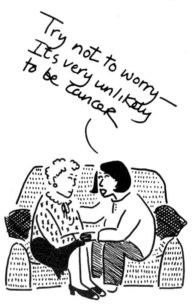

Rare forms of breast cancer There are a number of rare breast cancers. They have the same range of symptoms as more common cancers but have slightly different features. These can only be recognized under the microscope. They tend to grow more slowly and are less likely to spread.

Papillary breast cancer This grows in a similar way to a non-cancerous intraductal papilloma in an enlarged duct or cyst and is most likely to be found in the ducts beneath the nipple. About 2 per cent of breast cancers are papillary cancers.

Paget's disease Named after Sir James Paget who was the first to note that an underlying cancer in the breast can occasionally produce a skin rash in the nipple, similar to eczema. This crusty skin disorder may be the first indication of a cancer (non-invasive or invasive) which cannot yet be felt. Paget's disease accounts for about 2 per cent of breast cancers.

Medullary breast cancer This forms a well-defined lump with a capsule-like outer layer. For this reason it is sometimes called circumscribed carcinoma. Medullary cancers begin in the breast ducts. About 2 per cent of breast cancers are medullary cancers.

Mucinous breast cancer The cells of this cancer produce a mucus-like substance around the cancer cells. They account for about 1.5 per cent of breast cancers.

Tubular breast cancer So called because the cells form a tube-like pattern. There are some similarities with the cell formation of sclerosing adenosis. The tubule formation is sometimes combined with other cancer cells in the same growth. About 2 per cent of breast cancers are tubular.

Inflammatory breast cancer This produces the symptom of generalized inflammation in the breast. It is painful and extremely rare.

Checklist of symptoms and diseases

Most breast diseases share common symptoms and the same disease may produce slightly different symptoms in different women. A symptom is only an indication that something is wrong. The great majority will be due to minor problems and non-cancerous conditions.

Symptom	Possible problem/disease
Breast pain and tenderness (including the armpit)	Changing hormone levels in the monthly cycle; mastitis; abscess; cyst(s); fibroadenosis; sclerosing adenosis; fibrocystic disease; duct ectasia; fat necrosis; cancer (not often)
Breast lumps	Cyst; fibroadenoma; fibrous disease; intraductal papilloma; duct ectasia; lipoma; fat necrosis; cancer
Lumpiness and thickening in the breast	Changes in the monthly cycle; fibroadenosis; sclerosing adenosis; fibrocystic disease; cancer (not often)

Changes in breast size and shape	Changes in the monthly cycle; during pregnancy; large cyst and fibroadenoma; intraductal papilloma (occasionally); cancer
Inflammation in the breast	Mastitis; abscess; cyst (occasionally); intraductal papilloma (occasionally); duct ectasia; inflammatory cancer (very rare)
Changes in skin appearance and texture of breast	Irritation from clothing; detergents or cosmetics; skin rashes — eczema; abscess; duct ectasia; cancer
Dimpling of the skin	Intraductal papilloma (occasionally); duct ectasia; fat necrosis; cancer
Inverted nipples	Completely normal in women who have had inverted nipples since their breasts developed; sclerosing adenosis; intraductal papilloma (occasionally); duct ectasia; cancer
Nipple discharge	Due to hormone changes in the monthly cycle (nothing to worry about); during pregnancy (completely normal); overproduction of prolactin; mastitis; abscess; cyst (occasionally); fibrocystic disease; intraductal papilloma; duct ectasia; cancer
Enlarged lymph nodes	A complaint unrelated to the breasts; mastitis; abscess; duct ectasia; fat necrosis; cancer

Further reading

Michael Baum, *Breast Cancer: the facts* (Oxford University Press, 1988), briefly outlines different breast conditions, non-cancerous as well as cancerous (see Chapter 4).

Angela Phillips and Gill Rakusen, *Our Bodies — Our Selves* (Penguin Books, 1987), for general information about women's health.

CHAPTER FOUR
How breast problems come about

Breast problems arise when something goes wrong with the cells that make up breast tissue. To understand how different forms of treatment can help, we need to know about how cells reproduce themselves, what happens to them when something goes wrong, and how our immune system deals with cells that misbehave.

Cells in the human body

Cells are specialized — different types of cells perform different jobs. For example, some make up muscle, some carry oxygen (red blood cells), some fight disease (white blood cells). Cells perform different functions in our breasts.

Cell structure

Each cell is adapted in its size, shape and chemistry to the particular job it has to do. There is no such thing as a 'typical' cell, but all cells have common features. With a few exceptions they contain a nucleus, surrounded by cytoplasm. A thin flexible outer layer, the cell membrane, surrounds each cell.

The membrane surrounding each cell acts as a two way filter, controlling the substances that can enter and leave the cell. Nutrients (food) can pass into the cell. Nutrients provide energy. Some hormones provide instructions that cells need to do their specialized jobs.

The nucleus of each human cell contains DNA (deoxyribonucleic acid). DNA carries instructions, called genes, which tell the cell how to do its job. It provides the genetic blueprint which is needed for cells to grow and divide properly. DNA is designed to respond to hormone messages so that cell growth and development can take place.

How cells reproduce themselves

Cells have a limited life. When they wear out or die, or become damaged through injury or infection, new cells are needed to replace them. New cells are also necessary for growth.

Cell division (mitosis) Cells reproduce themselves by first growing and then dividing. This process is called mitosis. Normally cells only reproduce themselves if there is need for new or renewed tissue. Different types of cells wear out and need replacing at different rates. To maintain the renewal of tissue, the DNA of each cell contains instructions about how often the cell should divide, a sort of timer device. For example, skin cells and cells in the lining of the womb and gut divide more frequently, because they are easily worn away. Liver cells wear out more slowly and so divide much less frequently.

New cell growth (hyperplasia) The main times when new cell growth takes place in our breasts are during adolescence, when the breasts are developing, and during pregnancy when the breasts are getting ready to produce milk. This growth is triggered by hormones (see page 19). New cell growth may sometimes cause pain and lumpiness in the breasts.

Cells which misbehave

When a cell divides, every detail of the genetic code carried by the DNA is reproduced in the two new cells, including its built-in timer device and its ability to recognize hormone signals correctly.

Changes in cell behaviour

Minor irregularities in cell structure and behaviour happen all the time, but usually these are easily corrected or reversed. Such irregularities are described as metaplasia or dysplasia.

Unnecessary cell growth (neoplasia) If the instructions carried by DNA become significantly altered, either when a cell divides or when it's damaged, the normal features of cell behaviour can change. Alterations in the all-important timer mechanism can lead to new unnecessary cell growth.

Non-cancerous growths In cells which form benign, non-cancerous growths, the DNA coding has become altered, but most features of normal cell behaviour remain intact. Non-cancerous cells seem to be aware of their surroundings so don't overrun other healthy tissue.

Cancerous growth Cancerous growths are the result of more serious alterations in cell structure and behaviour, so that cells have sometimes changed beyond all recognition. Often they are no longer able to do their specialized job. Their timer device changes so that they tend to divide more frequently. They can overrun surrounding tissues and prevent healthy cells from thriving. Cancer cells also have a tendency to break off from the growth. They are then carried through the bloodstream and lymphatic system and may sometimes start cancerous growths (known as secondary cancers or metastases) elsewhere in the body.

Different forms of cancer

Cancer is a blanket term. There are many different forms of the disease. Some cancers can take 20 or 30 years to develop to the point where we notice them. Others develop much more rapidly. In some cancerous growths, cells begin to break off in the early stage of development. Others are much less likely to shed cells, and are therefore less serious.

Most cancers occur in epithelial cells. These are the cells which form the lining of external and internal body surfaces like the skin, the lungs, the gut, the womb and the lining of the ducts and lobules in the breast. Cancers which develop in epithelial cells are called carcinomas.

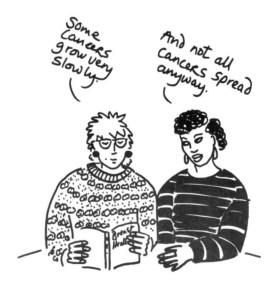

The cells which form the lining of the milk ducts and channels (see page 17) are influenced by hormonal messages throughout our reproductive lives. Some people think that this may affect the DNA in these cells in a way which increases the possibility of irregularities in cell growth.

Identifying cancerous cells

Most cancers can be distinguished from non-cancerous growths by their different cell structure. The technical term for differences in cell structure is differentiation. A 'well-differentiated' cell is one which has changed little from the normal structure of the original cell, whereas a 'poorly-differentiated' cell may have changed considerably. Differentiation is one of the factors which doctors look at when trying to assess the seriousness of breast cancer (see Chapter 15 for more information).

Precancerous cells Sometimes the dividing line between cancerous and non-cancerous cells is not clear. When abnormal cells are detected which seem to be neither one thing nor the other, they are usually described as precancerous. This means they may develop into cancer but many precancerous conditions remain precancerous and never develop further, sometimes clearing up without treatment.

If you have a breast lump, don't jump to conclusions

Remember that the great majority of breast lumps turn out to be non-cancerous and will never develop into cancer. If you are told you have a precancerous condition, this doesn't mean it will necessarily develop into cancer. If you are told you have breast cancer, bear in mind that this term covers different forms of cancer, some of which have a very good outlook.

The body's ability to heal itself

The body has its own natural defences which often enable it to heal itself when faced with illness or disease. This system of natural defences is called the immune system. It's helpful to understand how our immune system works and the part it can play in the control of disease, including cancer.

When we catch 'flu or get a throat infection, our bodies react. We may get a temperature, a sore throat or generally feel under the weather. These kinds of reactions to infections are the body's immune system working to correct the situation.

The immune system consists of groups of specialized cells, which have specific tasks in defending the body from illness. These specialized cells co-operate closely with each other. When bacteria or viruses enter the body, they are recognized as different from our own body cells. This is because cells display signals called antigens on their surface. When your immune system detects an unfamiliar antigen, it responds by attacking the unfamiliar cell, and usually destroys it.

The protective cells of the immune system are found in every part of our bodies. There are also stationary concentrations of some of these cells in the lymph nodes and spleen. They are able to trap and destroy foreign cells which get into the lymphatic system or bloodstream. Enlarged glands are often doing the work of protecting us against disease.

The immune system and cancer cells

Until recently it was thought that our immune system simply protected us from invading cells. It is now believed that the immune system can sometimes recognize and deal with abnormal changes in our own cells. Cancer cells probably occur in all of us throughout our lives but our immune system is normally able to detect and deal with these cells before they have a chance to develop into a cancerous growth. But in some circumstances our immune system appears to be overwhelmed. It is when this happens that cancer may develop.

We do not yet know why some cancer cells escape our body's immune system. Possibly these cells are able to disguise their antigen signal so that they are not detected by our natural defences. We also know that poor diet and stress can affect our immune system. When we are tired or under a lot of pressure at work, we are more likely to fall ill. As we get older too, our immune system tends to become less efficient. This is probably one reason why major illnesses, including cancer, occur in old age.

Medical scientists disagree about the importance of the immune system in dealing with cancer. Most think that the immune system is not strong enough to remove a cancer once it is large enough to be noticed. Others recognize that the health of the immune system is important in controlling the spread of the disease. They suggest that most of breakaway cells never have the chance to form secondary growths because the immune system destroys them first.

Treatments and their effects on the immune system

The main treatments for cancer offered by modern medicine are surgery, radiotherapy (using radiation) and drugs. All of them tend to affect the body's immune system as well as the cancer. The result is that these forms of treatment may weaken our body's own healing processes, (in the case of radiotherapy, for a long period of time after treatment has ended). Doctors argue that this is justified because these are the only treatments that can cure the disease or effectively control it.

Many of the traditional and complementary therapies discussed later in the book are concerned with ways of restoring or improving the body's self-healing abilities. Although doctors remain sceptical about this approach, some cancer sufferers have found these therapies have helped to counteract the unpleasant side-effects of modern treatments and, in some cases, have cured them of their disease. (You'll find more information about traditional and complementary treatments in Chapters 10 and 17.)

Further reading

John Cairns, *Cancer, Science and Society* (W.H. Freeman and Co, 1986), gives a detailed but highly technical explanation of cell processes which lead to different forms of cancer and looks at the methods used by Western science in understanding such processes (see Chapters 6, 7 and 8).

The Biology of Health and Disease (Open University Course 2055), includes a chapter on inflammation and immunity — quite complicated unless you have done some biology at school.

CHAPTER FIVE
What we know about the causes of breast disease

Any woman who discovers she has breast cancer is bound to ask herself: 'Why me?'

We don't yet know what causes breast cancer. Doctors and scientists have identified a number of factors which may influence the development of the disease, but there is no proof that any one factor actually *causes* breast cancer.

This chapter looks at some of the risks which have been identified. You may find it alarming to read about these risks — many of them are a part of our environment and our everyday lives — but remember that a risk is only an increased possibility. The great majority of women in any risk group *don't* get breast cancer.

We know little about the causes of non-cancerous breast conditions. Most doctors agree that these complaints are probably influenced by hormones because they mainly occur during our reproductive years and are affected by changes in the monthly cycle.

Most of the information in this chapter is about factors influencing breast cancer. Much less is known about non-cancerous conditions and so these are only mentioned if a particular study has identified a possible cause.

Cancer genes

Scientists have different theories about why some cells change when they reproduce themselves. One theory is that a cancer gene, called an 'oncogene', is present in the DNA spiral within cells. Some scientists think that this oncogene may lie dormant like a time-bomb until it is triggered into action by the natural ageing process or by some other factor.

What are the risks of getting breast cancer?

Breast cancer is the most common cancer affecting women (perhaps one reason why we fear it so much). Even so, it only affects one in twelve women. Eleven out of twelve women *don't* get the disease.

If a woman is exposed to certain risks, the chances of developing the disease increased. But a risk is *only* an increased possibility. It's worth bearing in mind that:

- the great majority of women in any risk group don't get breast cancer
- a woman affected by several risks does not necessarily develop breast cancer
- a woman who is apparently free from known risks may develop breast cancer.

Viruses

Some scientists think that a virus may interfere with the DNA blueprint in cells causing cancerous changes. Such a virus was identified in the milk of mice who developed breast cancer but as yet no virus has been found in human breast milk.

A study, by scientists at Liverpool University, identified a virus in the white blood cells of all but one of 32 women with breast cancer. A similar number of women without breast cancer were also tested. Only three were found to have the virus. This is strong evidence that a virus may be involved in breast cancer but the study points out that this is no proof that the virus *causes* breast cancer.

Radiation

Some forms of radiation occur naturally: sunlight, radon gas which seeps from the ground, and radiation from certain types of stone are examples. Other forms of radiation are manufactured: fallout from the testing of nuclear weapons and leakages from nuclear power plants for example. But radiation is also emitted from everyday household appliances such as televisions, computer screens, digital watches, clocks and radios. And radiation is widely used in medicine for X-rays and for radiotherapy. There are different types of radiation: high energy, ionizing radiation and low energy radiation.

High energy, ionizing radiation Ionizing radiation is a stream or ray of very high-energy particles which can enter and damage the genetic structure (the DNA) of living cells. Large doses of ionizing radiation are known to cause cancer. For example, the survivors of the atom bombs dropped on Hiroshima and Nagasaki showed a marked increase in all forms of cancer, including breast cancer, which was due to radiation fallout. Individuals accidentally exposed to even small doses of high energy radiation are more likely to develop some form of cancer, although this may happen twenty years or more after the event.

High energy radiation is used in the treatment of cancer. Radiotherapy is designed to damage and put out of action cancer cells using carefully controlled doses of ionizing radiation. (Although there is a slight risk of developing cancer from radiation treatment, most doctors argue that the benefits of treatment outweigh the possible danger involved.)

Low energy radiation Low energy radiation is far less likely to damage the DNA structure in cells. It's rather like the difference between using a bullet and a balloon to hit a target. What is not clear is whether large doses of low energy radiation, like continued use of a sun lamp or visual display unit, place people at risk. We do know that fair-skinned people who spend long hours in the sun are at some risk of developing skin cancer. Recent work at Harvard University has shown that multiple doses of low energy radiation may be at least as dangerous as one dose of high energy radiation.

Age

As we all know, ill health increases with age. It is not known whether this is because our bodies wear out and become less efficient at replacing cells, or because our immune system becomes less capable. Most cancers develop slowly, and it could be that the 'cause' happens many years earlier and it is only triggered into action later in life.

Age alone cannot be said to cause cancer. The incidence of breast cancer does increase with age, but the great majority of older women do not get the disease, and age does not explain why younger women in their thirties and forties develop it.

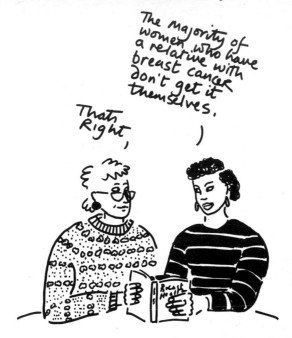

Family history

A woman has an increased risk of getting breast cancer if her mother, a sister or an aunt already has the disease. If the relative has cancer in both breasts, then her chances of getting breast cancer are further increased.

Scientists have looked to see if any genetic factor is responsible for this increased risk and there is some evidence this may be the case. Other doctors suggest that shared environmental factors such as social circumstance, diet, or patterns of stress in families may explain the increase in risk. Although there is an increased risk, the majority of women who have a relative with breast cancer don't get it themselves.

Reproductive history — our fertile years

Studies have shown that certain factors in our reproductive history (the pattern of our fertile years) appear to influence the possibility of breast cancer. Collecting this information is not easy since most women can't remember clearly when they started periods or when they stopped having them so it's difficult to judge whether research based on this kind of information is accurate.

Doctors have noticed that women who start their periods early, or who do not have children, or who stop having periods later in life than usual (a late menopause) are a little more likely to develop breast cancer. This suggests that the total number of periods in our fertile years may influence the likelihood of developing breast cancer (see 'Hormones', below). They've also noticed that women who have their children in their thirties and forties seem to be more likely to get breast cancer. It appears that having your children early, in your teens and early twenties has some protective effect.

Some studies suggest that breastfeeding gives protection against breast cancer but other studies find no clear evidence that this is so. There is evidence that breastfeeding may only give protection if it continues over years. For example there is a low incidence of breast cancer in Japan, where the average number of years spent breastfeeding is 6.4 years. This is also true for many other non-European and Third World countries where more than one child is breastfed over a number of years. But it is also possible that the low incidence of breast cancer in these countries is due not to breastfeeding but to other factors. More studies need to be done before we can say with certainty that breastfeeding for shorter periods (like the first few months after birth) gives us any protection.

The link between our reproductive years and non-cancerous breast disease is firmly established. The majority of these complaints occur during our child-bearing years and once the menopause has passed become increasingly rare. What is not clear is why some complaints (like fibroadenomas) are more likely in young women while others develop in the late thirties and forties (like cysts and fibrocystic disease).

Hormones

While hormones don't cause breast cancer, they seem to play a role in its development. The breast cells most likely to change and become cancerous are the cells which line the milk ducts and lobules. These cells are influenced by hormone signals throughout our reproductive years and it may make them open to abnormal changes. But we still know too little about hormones to say what role they might play in causing breast disease.

Hormone replacement therapy As well as naturally occurring changes in hormone levels during a woman's reproductive life, some women are given artificial hormones in the form of hormone replacement therapy (HRT), to lessen unpleasant symptoms of the menopause. The evidence about HRT is contradictory. Some studies suggest an increased risk of breast cancer in women who receive it, while others show little or no difference.

The Pill It may be another 10 or 20 years before we are able to study the long-term effects on women who have taken the contraceptive pill. Studies so far show an increased risk in women who started taking the Pill in their late teens or early twenties, or before their first pregnancy. Other studies suggest that long-term use of the Pill (8-12 years) may be a risk, particularly for women who used the earlier pills which contained higher doses of oestrogens. But there are also studies which suggest that the Pill may protect women from developing breast disease, both cancerous and non-cancerous breast conditions.

Nationality, race and class

Scientists who look at the possibility of environmental causes of breast cancer have investigated the pattern of the disease across different countries and cultures, and compared this with patterns of child-bearing, breastfeeding, diet and life-style. Many doctors are sceptical of the generalizations made on the basis of such studies because there are so many possible factors to look at and many possible explanations.

Nationality Britain has one of the highest rates of breast cancer of any country in the world where statistics are kept. It is closely followed by most of the industrialized countries (with the striking exception of Japan). Comparisons with less industrialized countries immediately show a marked contrast in the numbers of women developing breast cancer. Possible explanations include differences in diet and other factors, such as when women have children and the length of time they breastfeed.

Race Most scientists argue that the biological differences between humans are so superficial and so spread out and intermingled that it is meaningless to use the term 'race' to define biological groups. Studies which have looked at the incidence of breast cancer in different 'racial groups' (based on categories such as skin colour) have found no evidence that the disease is more likely in one group than another.

Variation in the risk of breast cancer in populations of different skin colour around the world is most likely to be due to cultural differences for example in diet, and in patterns of child rearing and breastfeeding — or to differences in the environment. One study looked at the risk of breast cancer among women of African origin in two different countries. It found that 58 in every 1,000 black women in the San Francisco Bay area of the United States are likely to develop breast cancer, compared with only 14 in every 1,000 in Bulawayo, Zimbabwe.

Ethnic origin Some studies have also looked at how migration of an ethnic group to a new country affects the chances of developing breast cancer. They have found that granddaughters of migrant women who are born in the country of settlement have the same chance of developing the disease as any other women in the population. We don't know whether this is due to things like changes in diet, or patterns in child-rearing, or to other factors not yet identified.

Class It is difficult to separate the effects of race and class because most black people are found in working-class jobs and live in working-class areas.

We would expect to find a greater risk of disease among working-class women because of factors such as diet, stress, poor working or housing conditions and poorer access to medical facilities. Many diseases follow this pattern in our society (cervical cancer, another cancer in women, is particularly related to class). Breast cancer, however, seems to be an exception, with a higher percentage of upper- and middle-class women developing the disease. It is thought that this may be because working-class women tend to start their families younger than middle-class women. Some groups of ethnic origin in the working class also have less animal fats in their diet.

More studies need to be done if we are to have a clearer understanding of race and class differences in the possibility of developing breast cancer.

Diet

In Britain, along with most industrialized countries, we eat a diet rich in meat and dairy products, and we consume large quantities of sugar and refined foods such as white bread. We tend to eat few fresh vegetables, fruits or different types of beans, grains and pulses, which are a major source of fibre. These fibre-rich foods form the staple diet in most African, Asian and Latin American countries.

There are two ways in which scientists explore the links between diet and breast cancer. One approach, already mentioned, looks at the statistics on breast cancer in different countries and cultures, drawing a general picture of how they relate to different dietary habits. The second approach tests various food-stuffs on animals, generally in large doses, to see whether they produce cancerous changes.

Both approaches have shortcomings. Cross-cultural comparisons between countries and peoples tend to be too general to pinpoint specific foods. Establishing a link between diet and breast cancer is by no means the same as proving that one causes the other. Food experiments with animals are also questionable as human responses to food-stuffs may be quite different from the animals tested.

Despite these limitations, there is a growing body of evidence linking the foods we eat (and perhaps the foods we don't eat) with the development of cancer.

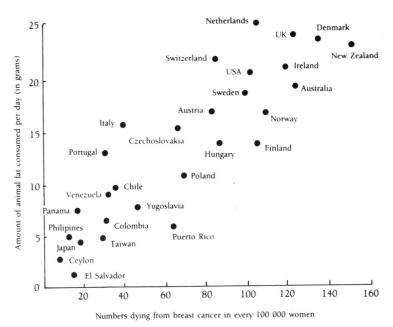

Figure 5 Comparison of animal fat consumption and breast cancer in different countries (From Experimental Evidence in Dietary Factors and Dependent Cancers, *K. Carroll.)*

Fats Countries where fat consumption is high, have high breast cancer rates, and the reverse is true for countries where fat consumption is low. Experimental studies on animals seem to bear out these conclusions.

It is not clear why fats and oils might have this effect. One possibility is that fats reduce the immune system's ability to clear away any abnormal cells, increasing the chance of cancer developing, or it may be that women who have had a high fat diet, particularly in their youth, have higher levels of oestrogen released from fat cells which may promote cancer after the change of life.

One problem with these studies is that it is difficult to isolate the effects of fats from other elements in our diet. Critics argue that the statistics linking fat consumption to breast cancer could equally apply to the consumption of meat, or to the total number of calories in our diet (see comments on weight, page 48).

Sugar A study covering 21 countries showed a possible link between sugar consumption (including syrup, molasses, honey and sugary foods) and the increased likelihood of breast cancer. We don't know why this should be. One suggestion is that high sugar levels lead to higher levels of insulin in the bloodstream, which has a similar effect on breast tissue to oestrogen and progesterone. Another possibility is that the body uses excess sugar to make more oestrogen.

Coffee A number of studies have noted a link between coffee consumption and non-cancerous breast disease. In particular, fibrocystic disease and fibroadenosis seem to be affected by levels of caffeine.

Strangely, caffeine may have a beneficial effect for women who have breast cancer. One study found that cell differentiation improved in women with breast cancer who drank several cups of coffee a day. (More information about cell differentiation can be found in Chapter 4.) No studies have found that caffeine consumption protects women from developing breast cancer, and these findings of improved cell differentiation need to be confirmed by other studies.

Alcohol

A number of studies suggest that drinking alcohol may increase the possibility of getting breast cancer. Even moderate drinking of beers, wines and spirits (up to three drinks a day) may have this effect. However, as with other foods and drinks, it is difficult to single out alcohol from all the other aspects of our lives which may influence our chances of developing breast cancer.

Weight

Overeating and overweight are linked with breast cancer in post-menopausal women. This may be because fat cells release oestrogen, raising oestrogen levels in the body. It is possible that overweight is *the* factor linking diet and breast cancer.

Smoking

Although smoking has been linked to a number of different cancers, including cervical cancer, no link has been established between smoking and breast cancer.

Stress, personality and circumstance

Stress has been linked with cancer because it has been noticed that people who develop cancer have often suffered some great upset or distress in their lives in the months or years leading up to cancer. This has led scientists to consider the possible effects of stress on the immune system. It is thought that stress makes the immune system less efficient. The specialized cells which stop cancer developing (known as natural killer cells or macrophages), seem to be particularly affected by increased levels of stress, lowering our defences against disease.

A similar line of enquiry has looked at the ways in which we react to and cope with illness. Some studies have shown that women with determination and women who deny that anything is wrong tend to respond better to treatment than women who feel overwhelmed and defeated by their illness. This has led some scientists to speculate that some personality types may be more prone to developing cancer than others. They suggest that people who bottle up or deny their feelings are more likely to develop cancer.

There is a danger with these studies of drawing over-simple conclusions on the basis of very uncertain evidence. What we do know is that stress affects our ability to heal ourselves — to say more than this is probably unwise.

Non-cancerous breast disease

You may be afraid if you have a breast problem that it is likely to turn into breast cancer. This is not the case. The great majority of non-cancerous breast conditions remain non-cancerous. There is an increased risk in a small percentage of non-cancerous conditions where the cell changes are unusual. (This only occurs in about 4 per cent of non-cancerous breast conditions.)

What conclusions can we draw?

All the factors we have looked at shed some light on the possible causes of breast cancer and non-cancerous breast disease but none of them gives a complete answer.

With so many different factors at work, it would be wrong to single out any particular 'risk' and allow it to determine our life-choices. We must not forget that the great majority of women will not get breast cancer or any other breast disease. Rather than let the fear of cancer overwhelm us, we can use the information in this chapter to try and improve our health and self-healing capacity by taking steps to minimize the risks over which we have some control.

Further reading

Michael Baum, *Breast Cancer: The Facts* (Oxford University Press, 1988), looks at causes of breast cancer in Chapter 2.

John Cairns, *Cancer, Science and Society* (W. H. Freeman and Co., 1986), gives a general outline of the causes of different kinds of cancer (see Chapters 3 and 4). This book is thorough but very technical.

CHAPTER SIX

What we can do for ourselves

Many breast problems can be helped by simple things which we can do for ourselves. This chapter explores ways of looking after our breasts from day to day, and the steps we can take to help prevent problems in pregnancy and breastfeeding. Often breast health is closely related to our overall health and well-being so some suggestions are specific to our breasts and others are about our general health.

Examining our breasts is a simple way of checking for any changes in them. This chapter explains how to examine your breasts and the best time to do it. It's worth bearing in mind that breast self-examination doesn't suit all women — it can cause some of us unnecessary anxiety. The arguments for and against breast self-examination are explained so that each woman can decide for herself.

Day-to-day breast care

Breast pain and discomfort can affect our lives in many ways.

> For a week before my period, my breasts get really swollen and lumpy. I'm conscious of them the whole time.

> When I get overtired or have a bad time at work my breasts feel all tender, like swollen glands.

Most women put up with problems because their symptoms come and go and in the meantime they get on with their busy lives. Looking after our breasts means looking after ourselves as women. Here are some things we can do to improve our general health, which will also help to ease breast pain and discomfort and prevent problems developing:

Choosing the right bra. If you wear a bra, make sure your bra supports your breasts *and* is comfortable to wear. Choosing a bra on the basis of how big a cleavage it gives you may put pressure on tender breast tissue, making you ache. Bras which have a rigid plastic frame for support can dig into the underside of the breast causing pain. An elasticated border crossing your breasts may be the culprit so it's important to give yourself enough time to choose a bra which will suit *your* breasts and be comfortable to wear.

If you have large or floppy breasts, a bra is an important support and may need to be worn at night if you get breast pain. This helps to stop the weight of the breast pulling as you turn over in bed.

Comfortable clothes. Check that your clothes don't drag across your breasts either because they are tight-fitting or because they get trapped by the way you are lying at night. The secret is to make sure your clothes are comfortable during the day and in bed at night.

Good posture can help. If you tend to slump forward and crowd your breasts together, perhaps because you sit down at work all day, you may find this causes you pain. Simple breathing exercises, to expand your lungs and give your breasts enough space can help. Some women find yoga exercises useful for good breathing and improving posture and balance.

Getting rid of tension and fatigue. Sometimes tension or tiredness can increase breast tenderness, particularly in the part of the breast which reaches up into the armpit. A good rest helps, but this depends on whether you are able to relax. There are a number of simple relaxation exercises which you can do, sitting in a chair at work or at home, or lying down, maybe before you go to bed. (A relaxation exercise is given on page 155.)

Diet can help to relieve swollen breasts. Many women's breasts become enlarged before a period because of fluid retention in the tissue. The swelling can be painful. Some foods increase the possibility of fluid retention while other foods help to minimize it. Having a varied diet including fresh fruit and vegetables, cutting down (or cutting out) tea, coffee and salt and reducing animal fats all help to give you a healthier diet and reduce fluid retention. Foods which help to reduce fluids building up are cucumber, parsley, grapefruit, apples, potatoes and white grapes.

Exercise is good for you. Regular exercise is important for your general health. It helps to release tension, and tones up your body tissue. You can start getting fitter by choosing just one exercise activity and building on that. For example you might go for a walk in your lunch hour, go swimming once a week, or go to a keep-fit class. Some women find it helpful to do breast exercises for a few minutes every night and morning.

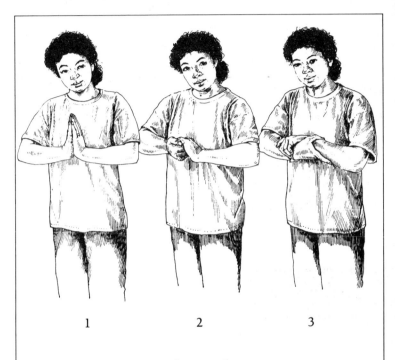

1   2   3

Figure 6 Three simple exercises

1 *Press the palms of your hands together in front of your breasts*

2 *Gripping your hands together in front of your breasts, pull your fingers away from each other*

3 *Grasping your forearms in front of your breasts, pull your arms away from each other*

You may need to lose some weight. Excess weight can contribute to breast pain and discomfort by increased breast size and breast weight. Dieting is often easier if it is combined with regular exercise.

These common-sense measures can help to minimize breast problems and improve your general health. But if pain, tenderness, swelling or any other symptom continues, then seek professional help. Chapters 8, 9 and 10 discuss ways of doing this.

Breast care during pregnancy and breastfeeding

Most of the suggestions above apply equally to pregnancy and breastfeeding. Sore or cracked nipples and mastitis often begin because a mother isn't able to rest enough or is too busy to sit down and eat a proper meal. There are a number of things you can do to help to prevent problems arising.

● One way of helping to prevent sore or cracked nipples is to prepare the nipples before birth by gently rubbing them with a flannel or towel when you wash. Also dressing without a bra for a few hours each day in the last weeks of pregnancy can help to 'toughen' your nipples in readiness for breastfeeding.

● Try gently pulling the nipple out and roll it between your finger and thumb, using a small amount of baby oil or cream. This helps to strengthen the nipple and is particularly helpful if you have an inverted nipple. It should be done with care to avoid any bruising. Your doctor may suggest other gentle exercises to help the nipple to stand out. She may also advise you to wear a small breast shield during pregnancy and breastfeeding, which has the same effect.

● Don't use soap on your nipples when you wash yourself during pregnancy and breastfeeding. Soap dries up the natural oils in the nipples. These oils help to protect your nipples against soreness or cracking.

● Making sure that your nipples are dry after feeding or washing helps to prevent soreness and infection. This means changing a bra or nursing pad if it becomes wet.

● If you feel your nipples are becoming sore, expose them to sunlight and air for a few minutes each day.

● Make sure you have a healthy diet and as much rest and relaxation as possible in the last weeks of pregnancy and while you are breastfeeding.

You'll find more information about how to treat sore nipples and other complaints related to breastfeeding in Chapter 11.

Checking your breasts for problems

The checklist on page 31 shows that many breast complaints share the same symptoms. This is important to remember when you examine your breasts so that you don't jump to the conclusion that you have cancer if you find a change in them. The aim of breast self-examination is for you to detect any change in your breasts as early as possible so that you have a greater choice of treatment and a better chance of a speedy recovery. This is as true for an abscess or a papilloma as it is for breast cancer.

Regular breast self-examination allows you to know your breasts better. Maybe one is larger than the other or is placed lower on the chest. Maybe you have one nipple which is inverted or turned in or maybe you have had lumpy breasts for many years. Sometimes clothing tends to bring you up in a rash in the area of your breasts. Only if you examine your breasts regularly will you know if anything has changed which should be checked.

Many changes take place in our breasts during our adult lives. If you discover anything unusual, don't fear the worst. Remember that the great majority of breast problems, including breast lumps, are *not* cancerous.

There are many leaflets which explain breast self-examination — a list is given at the end of this chapter. The following information comes from a leaflet produced by the Health Education Authority.

How to examine your breasts

The best time to examine your breasts is just after a period, when your breasts are usually softest and no longer tender. Or, if you've stopped having periods, choose a day in the month you'll be able to remember, like the first day or the last. The important thing is to examine your breasts regularly, at the same time each month.

Breast self-examination

There are two stages to examining your breasts. The first is looking and the second is feeling. When you examine your breasts you are trying to detect anything that is *unusual* or anything that is different from last time. For this, looking is just as important as feeling.

Looking

Undress to the waist and sit or stand in front of a mirror in a good light. (You may prefer to do this in the morning before you get dressed or last thing at night.) When you look at your breasts, remember that no two are the same — not even your own two.

First, let your arms hang loosely by your sides and look at your breasts in the mirror.

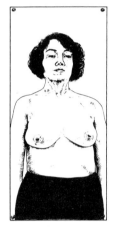

Here's what to look for:

- Any change in the size of either breast
- Any change in either nipple
- Bleeding or discharge from either nipple
- Any unusual dimple or puckering on the breast or nipple
- Veins standing out more than is usual for you

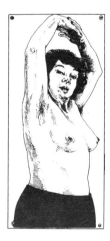

Next raise your arms above your head. Watch in the mirror as you turn from side to side to see your breasts from different angles.

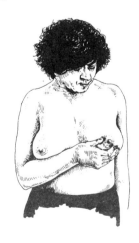

Now look down at your breasts and squeeze each nipple gently to check for any bleeding or discharge that is unusual for you.

Feeling

Lie down on your bed and make yourself comfortable with your head on a pillow. Examine one breast at a time.

Put a folded towel under your shoulder blade on the side you are examining. This helps to spread the breast tissue so that it is easier to examine.

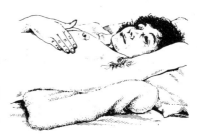

Use your right hand to examine your left breast and vice versa. Put the hand you are not using under your head.

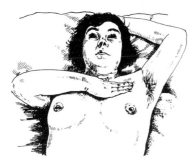

Keep your fingers together and use the flat of the fingers, not the tips.

Start from the collarbone above your breast.

Trace a continuous spiral round your breast moving your fingers in small circles. Feel gently but firmly for any unusual lump or thickening.

Work round the outside of your breast first. When you get back to your starting point work round again in a slightly smaller circle and so on. Keep on doing this until you have worked right up to the nipple. Make sure you cover every part of your breast.

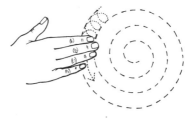

You may find a ridge of firm tissue in a half-moon shape under your breast. This is quite normal. It is tissue that develops to help support your breast.

Finally examine your armpit. Still use the flat of your fingers and the same small circular movements to feel for any lumps.

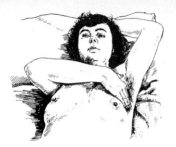

Start right up in the hollow of your armpit and gradually work down towards your breast.

It is important not to forget this last part of the examination.

If you think you've found something unusual in one breast but you're not sure, check the same part of the other breast. If both breasts feel the same, it's probably just the way your breasts are made.

If you still think something may be wrong, then see your doctor. It doesn't matter how uncertain you are. It's far better to see your doctor and set your mind at rest than risk neglecting something serious.

Make a note of where the lump or change is. Arrange to see your doctor within the next few days. In the meantime, try not to keep feeling the lump to see if it has gone away or got any bigger. It's best to leave it alone. *Remember, most lumps are not cancerous.*

Some leaflets also tell you to report any odd feelings of discomfort or pain in one breast. While it is important to note any change, pain and discomfort are extremely common in women's breasts and they are not usually a symptom of cancer.

Supporters and critics of breast self-examination

Supporters of breast self-examination (BSE) argue that women who regularly check for themselves are likely to find cancerous lumps earlier than women who don't. And smaller lumps have a better overall outlook. The problem is that the evidence supporting this is mixed. Some early detection campaigns using breast self-examination have detected no more early cancers than in the population at large. Critics of BSE argue that education campaigns for breast self-examination lead to increased anxiety in women who either dread examining themselves each month or who feel guilty because they can't face examining their breasts. Until there is clear evidence that BSE leads to the early detection and successful treatment of breast cancer, critics feel that such worry and preoccupation is unjustified.

> What I wind myself up about is self-examination. I know all the women's health books tend to do it but I don't because I just find ribs and things and I panic.

If you find the idea of breast self-examination too threatening or you are worried that you are not doing it correctly, contact your doctor, community nurse, well-woman clinic or family planning clinic who can check your breasts for you or teach you how to do it properly. The important thing is not to get unduly worried.

> It was making me neurotic. I'm sure it is a good thing for other people to do but it was making me feel lumps where there weren't any. I was pleased to hand the responsibility to someone else. I now go for six-monthly check-ups at the hospital.

Traditional and complementary therapies

Several of the traditional and complementary therapies described later in this book include treatments which we can do for ourselves. Some of these include diet, massage, exercise, water therapy and techniques for reducing stress and tension. You'll find more information about these in Chapters 10 and 17.

Further reading

Dorothy Brewster, *You can breast feed your baby . . . even in special situations* (Rodale Press, 1979).

Maire Messenger Davies, *The Breastfeeding Book*, (Century Paperbacks, 1982).

Angela Phillips and Jill Rakusen, *Our Bodies, Our Selves (Penguin, 1987)*.

BUPA *How to examine your breasts.*

Health Education Authority, *A guide to examining your breasts.*

Nottingham Breast Screening Unit, *Breast self-examination.*

Royal Marsden Hospital, Patient Education Group, *Breast self-examination.*

Tenovus Cancer Information Centre, Cardiff, *Breast self-examination,* and *Taking care of yourself.*

Women's National Cancer Control Campaign, *Everyone's doing the breast test,* and *Your life in your hands.*

CHAPTER SEVEN

Different approaches to health and disease

This chapter looks at different approaches to health and disease. It considers different health choices open to us. It looks at the advances made by modern medicine and considers some of its limitations. It also explains how modern treatments are tested. It then considers other systems of medicine practised in the world together with several complementary therapies which are available in this country. The chapter ends by suggesting that we need to learn to be assertive about our choices when we're talking to health professionals.

The advances and limitations of modern medicine

The system of medicine most widely practised in Britain is based on the different disciplines of western science. (It is sometimes called 'scientific medicine', 'technological medicine' or 'western medicine'.) In this book it will be called modern medicine.

Developments over the last 150 years

Modern medicine has changed considerably over the last century and a half as new scientific discoveries have been made in Europe and the United States. The study of cells was unheard of before the invention of high powered microscopes and the development of biochemistry. Antibiotics and vaccines have helped to wipe out a number of infectious diseases although some argue that improvements in diet and housing have been equally important. New advances have been made in surgical techniques such as open heart and transplant surgery. The twentieth century has also seen the development of a wide range of manufactured drugs to treat many illnesses. One of the most important steps in making modern medicine widely available in Britain was the setting up of a 'free' National Health Service by the Labour government after the Second World War.

Emphasis on physical symptoms These advances have not been without their limitations. Modern medicine's emphasis on scientific method has meant that health care has concentrated on the diagnosis and treatment of the *physical* symptoms of disease. These can be analysed, tested and measured with great precision. Modern medicine is not so good at assessing how our emotional, psychological and social well-being influences our health and little progress has been made in the field of mental illness.

'High-tech' medicine Modern medicine has developed a highly sophisticated technology. Many women first come across this when they have their babies in hospital. High-tech medicine can be frightening and leave the patient unsure of what is happening and why.

Large institutions like hospitals tend to be impersonal and many patients feel they are part of a production-line. Health professionals can easily slip into identifying individuals by their disease or symptoms.

> At the hospital, they have this fixed thing about you being a breast. 'Ah yes. You're the subcutaneous, aren't you?' And the students were coming in and saying 'Oh, we've not seen one of these. Can we have a look at it?'

A problem arises with increased specialization by doctors in modern medicine. Some patients see several different doctors in the course of one stay in hospital. While it is argued that this gives the patient the best treatment available, it can lead to a lack of communication between doctors and patients. Many hospital doctors find that their field of knowledge is so specialized that it is not easy to explain the complexities of a problem. They are under such pressure at work that often their only knowledge of a patient is a set of hospital notes handed to them before they see the patient. The lack of relationship between patient and doctor makes it difficult for patients to ask questions or express their fears.

Many health professionals are themselves concerned that these advances in technology and specialization make it increasingly difficult for most patients to understand what is wrong with them or understand what is happening when they seek treatment.

Other critics voice concern about the treatments offered by modern medicine. Many of these treatments require hospitalization and specialist care and many have unpleasant or serious side-effects.

It is also argued that modern medicine's emphasis on treating the symptoms of disease has meant that preventive medicine and the wider issues of whole-person health care have been neglected. Most people see their doctors when they become ill; they aren't encouraged to consult their GP about staying healthy. Some GPs try to bridge the gap by offering health screening for older patients, well-woman clinics, classes in relaxation, diet, giving up smoking, etc. But these opportunities are still not widely available and the present lack of funding for the Health Service means that health education and preventive medicine will continue to compete with other pressing needs.

Clinical trials

Modern medicine tests each treatment over years using large numbers of patients. Different treatments are carefully compared to see if one has any advantages over another already existing treatment. (This is how doctors know that, in many cases, lumpectomy with radiotherapy is as effective as mastectomy for treating primary breast cancer — see Chapter 12.) All trials use a strict procedure so that no bias enters into the results.

Clinical trials can interfere with women's choices because some hospitals will be testing one form of treatment at the expense of others. In theory women should be told if they are taking part in a trial and given the choice to refuse, but in practice it's tempting for doctors to neglect to inform their patients about trial studies. Their advice, and the information they give, can be influenced by their interest in establishing new treatments.

Running clinical trials is an important way of testing treatments but it is equally important that women are fully informed about their choices.

Traditional systems of health care

There are a number of traditional medical systems in different parts of the world which reach back thousands of years before modern scientific discoveries. Traditional systems of medicine are widely practised in China, Japan, the Indian subcontinent and among the native Indians of North and South America. Many other local systems of health care are used in different communities in the world.

In many countries traditional medicine exists alongside modern medicine but separate from it. Only in a few countries (e.g. China, Vietnam and parts of India) have governments actively encouraged co-operation between modern and traditional medicine and attempted to establish a state system of health care which provides both.

Whole-person framework

What most systems of traditional medicine have in common is a holistic framework which makes no clear division between the individual's physical, mental and emotional well-being. Health and disease are explained in terms of balance or imbalance of natural forces and life-giving energy. Human health is placed within a cosmic framework in which the individual's state of mind, social relationships and whole way of life are believed to have as much influence on their state of health as bacteria, viruses or other causes of illness which can be scientifically established. The practice of good health is seen as a way of life.

Self-healing

Great emphasis is placed on self-healing and the participation of the individual in getting well and staying well. The professional health worker is there to advise and support but each person is encouraged to take responsibility for their own health. Treatment sometimes provides a valuable form of psychotherapy, suggesting ways of changing the individual's approach to life.

All traditional systems have their own theories about health, illness and treatment but the types of treatment used are often similar. These include diet, herbal remedies, breathing exercises, massage, physical exercise, mental relaxation and healing rituals.

Complementary therapies

The word complementary comes from the verb to complete. Complementary therapies have grown up more recently with the development of modern medicine, for example, homoeopathy and naturopathy. They see themselves as providing an alternative to many of the high-tech treatments used by modern medicine. Like traditional medicines, they start from a whole-person standpoint and seek to restore a health giving 'balance' in the life of the person concerned.

Complementary therapies often fill in the gaps in treatment offered by modern medicine — where some treatments are under-financed and not considered a priority in the present climate of cost-effective health care. These include counselling and psychotherapy, art and music therapy, people qualified in relaxation techniques, massage, diet, nutritional medicine and a number of other health related practices.

Criticisms of alternative medicine

Unscientific A major stumbling block in understanding many traditional and complementary systems of medicine is that their explanations of health and illness have no meaning in a western scientific framework. There is no evidence of a vital force or flow of energy which can be measured or viewed under a microscope. While modern drugs are carefully tested and examined to treat particular symptoms, traditional remedies appear vague and unconvincing. The British Medical Association argues that the majority of alternative and complementary medicines should be dismissed as unsound. They suggest that if people benefit from any treatment, it's because the person believes in it not because the treatment itself works.

Responsibility for illness Critics are concerned that the idea of 'personal responsibility' can lead to people feeling guilty and ashamed: 'It's my fault that I'm ill' or 'It's my fault I'm not getting better'. They argue that personal responsibility for health doesn't take into account the many economic and social factors which are largely out of our control.

Standards of training and practice Modern medicine is also critical of the lack of training standards leading to recognized qualifications. Although professional bodies do exist to monitor training and standards in traditional and complementary medicine (see address list on page 192), anyone can set up as a private health practitioner without registering with any of these bodies. This can lead to abuses. Critics suggest that vulnerable people are conned and waste their money on useless remedies.

This problem cannot be resolved while only one model of medicine, based on western science, is officially accepted. Several alternative and complementary health bodies have applied for permission to practise within the health service but none have been admitted, apart from homoeopathy.

Closing the gap

In spite of the gap between modern medicine and alternative

approaches, there has been increasing contact and co-operation in the past few years. The work of alternative health clinics and specialists has been publicized in the media. Recent scientific research has suggested that diet, stress and relaxation may play a far more significant role in our health than was previously thought. Research into how the immune system works is still very new. But there is some evidence that self-healing plays an important role in coping with disease.

All health professions are increasingly recognizing the principle of 'holistic health care'. For some, this means improving the quality of care within the NHS. For others, it means recognizing the value of alternative approaches and working more closely with alternative practitioners. But it may be some time before the principles of whole-person health care become widespread in NHS practice. In the meantime women who want whole-person health care may have to choose a combination of different therapies (see Chapters 10 and 17).

Our right to health

It was suggested earlier that some doctors feel their patients are incapable of understanding what is wrong with them and pressure of work means little attempt is made to educate them. This lack of communication often leads to a lack of democracy: the doctor knows best and therefore she makes the decisions.

It is very difficult for women to challenge this situation. We often feel at a disadvantage speaking to doctors if we are half-clothed or lying in bed. Most doctors are men and many women don't feel confident talking to them about sensitive areas of their health. This leaves many women feeling that they have no control over what is happening to them in hospital or in the surgery.

Traditional and complementary practitioners should be more approachable and more committed to our active participation in the diagnosis and treatment of disease, but this may not always be so. Barriers of authority and insensitivity to women's feelings can still be present.

We should never forget that health professionals are providing a *service* which we pay for through taxes or direct charges. We are entitled to be treated with dignity and sensitivity if we seek their help. It's not always easy to find the confidence to ask for information, to voice any worries or fears and to take decisions about our health and the treatments offered to us. Being ill makes us feel vulnerable and it can be difficult enough to hang on to our dignity, let alone assert our rights. But it can help to keep these rights clearly in view. Here is a charter; write it down, look at it when you are waiting for an appointment and repeat it to yourself when you need confidence:

● We have the right to be treated with respect as intelligent, adult people

● We have the right to information about our health, about our diagnosis or treatment and about the side-effects of treatment

● We have the right to express our feelings and our worries about any aspect of our health

● We have the right to refuse any treatment we're not happy with

● We have the right to change our minds in the light of new information.

Further reading

Anne Dickson, *A woman in your own right — assertiveness and you* (Quartet Books, 1988).

Carolyn Faulder, *Whose body is it? The troubling issue of informed consent* (Virago, 1985).

Stephen Fulder, *How to Survive Medical Treatment — A holistic approach to the risks and side-effects of orthodox medicine* (Century Paperbacks, 1987).

Brian Inglis, *The Diseases of Civilisation — why we need a new approach to medical treatment* (Granada Publishing Ltd, 1983).

Brian Inglis and Ruth West, *The Alternative Health Guide* (Michael Joseph, 1983).

Dr. Andrew Stanway, *Alternative Medicine — A guide to natural therapies* (Penguin, 1986).

British Medical Association Board of Science Report on Alternative Therapies, May, 1986. This is expensive to buy but can be obtained through your public library. It uses technical language and is difficult to read but important in understanding modern medicine's criticisms of traditional and complementary medicine.

The British Holistic Medical Association Report on the BMA Board of Science Report, July, 1986. This is also expensive and quite difficult to read but gives a useful reply to the BMA report.

CHAPTER EIGHT
Going to see the doctor

If you are worried by a 'change' in your breasts, you may want to seek help from your doctor or a local clinic. If anxiety and fear about cancer stop you going remember that no health problem is too small or insignificant to be overlooked. Your doctor is there to help you to find out what is wrong and put your mind at ease.

This chapter tells you what to expect when you go to the doctor. It explains the procedure if your doctor thinks you need to have a further examination or test in the hospital. It also looks at other clinics and breast screening facilities which are available in different parts of the country.

Some women may not be happy with the way they are treated by their doctor or the consultant they see in outpatients. This chapter, therefore, explains how to change your doctor or consultant, if you need to, and how to have a say in deciding which hospital you will go to, if your doctor thinks it necessary. It also explains what to do if you feel you have been treated badly by a doctor and wish to make a complaint.

Going to the doctor or attending a hospital appointment when you have a breast problem can be quite an ordeal. Most women are preoccupied by the worry of breast cancer and many women find that they come away feeling that they didn't ask the right questions or didn't feel they had any control over the situation. This chapter gives some practical suggestions about how to cope with these interviews with doctors.

What to expect at the surgery

Your doctor may start by asking you some questions about your general health and what you think is wrong. She may want to know some details about your reproductive history such as when you started your periods, whether your periods are regular, if you have had any children and what part of the monthly cycle you are in. She will ask you about the menopause, whether you are on the Pill or are having hormone replacement therapy. She may ask if there is any history of breast disease in the family.

Personal questions like this can be disconcerting. It may be a good idea to think about them beforehand and come prepared with the necessary information. You may also like a friend or relative to be with you during the interview. Your own doctor may know the answers to some of these questions but another doctor in the practice or a hospital doctor will know very little and will want to check any written information she has received.

The doctor will examine your breasts using the same procedure as for breast self-examination (see Chapter 6). She will look at the appearance of the breasts and nipples and then carefully feel the breasts for any lumps or thickening. She may ask you which breast is causing problems and then start by examining the other breast in order to make a comparison. (The technical name for feeling the breasts is palpation. A lump which you can feel is called a palpable lump.)

Your GP may only see 15 to 20 women each year who come with a breast lump or other symptom and so has little experience of examining breasts for abnormalities. Most GPs don't have the equipment or skills to take a sample of breast tissue (see Chapter 9 on hospital tests). Usually, your doctor will refer you to hospital, but this does not necessarily mean something is wrong.

The family planning or well-woman clinic

If you don't feel confident enough to go to your own doctor with a breast problem, you can go to a family planning clinic or well-woman clinic for a breast examination. Your Community Health Council (in the phone book) will tell you where your nearest clinic is. There is usually a woman doctor whom you can ask to see if this is important to you. Family planning clinics and well-woman clinics will have more experience of breast examination but they are not always able to refer you to hospital for tests. This is usually done through your GP.

Making an appointment at the hospital

Your GP will make an appointment by sending a letter to a

particular consultant at a hospital in your area. They will arrange for you to attend an outpatient clinic. This usually takes less than a week but occasionally it may be longer. Waiting can be a time of great anxiety.

> I felt so anxious, I couldn't bear to be alone.

What your doctor says can make a difference to how you feel.

> I wasn't too worried. My doctor said she thought it was probably nothing but it was better to make sure.

Unfortunately some doctors are careless in the way they talk to patients about going to hospital. Many women leave their GPs surgery convinced they've got cancer. This is not the case. Tests and X-rays in hospital are routine. A very small percentage of women referred to hospital turn out to have cancer.

The outpatient clinic

You may be referred to a breast clinic or to a surgical outpatients clinic. Your GP will have made an appointment for you to see a consultant. A consultant is a doctor with considerable experience in a particular area. Your consultant will be a surgeon who has experience of breast surgery, although this may not be his main area of expertise. Consultants have one or two doctors working closely with them called registrars. You may see either the consultant or a registrar. Sometimes junior doctors or medical students are also present.

Waiting Waiting in outpatients can be nerve-racking, particularly if there is a delay. You could take something to read to take your mind off things. Taking a relative or a friend is a good idea if you want company while you're waiting. You can also take someone with you into the consultation if you'd like moral support when you see the doctor.

> My friend, who had experienced breast problems, came with me. Doctors use so many different terms and there seemed to be so much to remember that it helped having someone who knew something about it. We discussed it afterwards when I was calmer and compared notes about what the doctor had said and what we thought she had meant.

Seeing the hospital doctor The hospital doctor will start by asking you questions similar to those your doctor asks. This may

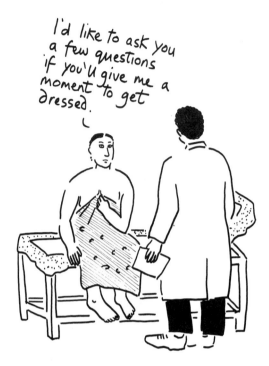

be in the consultant's office or in a private interview room where you can sit and discuss what you think may be wrong. You will then be asked to undress to the waist in a cubicle and wait for the doctor to examine you. The cubicle will contain a bed and possibly some hooks for your clothes and a wash basin. You may be given a sheet to cover yourself while you wait for the doctor.

The hospital doctor will again examine your breasts. After the examination, the doctor will discuss with you the need for any tests or X-rays (see Chapter 9).

Lying on a bed, stripped to the waist, with the doctor standing over you isn't the best situation to be in to have a discussion about possible tests or treatment. It is difficult to feel in control of the situation. Your consultant or registrar should allow you time to sit up and dress or cover yourself before discussing with you any tests he might recommend. In this way you will be in a better position to decide if you want any tests and which ones you want. Don't be afraid to take the initiative when the examination has finished. Sit up and say something like 'I'd like to ask you some questions if you'll just give me a moment to get dressed.'

It can be helpful to write down what you want to ask on a piece of paper. Most doctors react very positively to patients who do this and will take the time to answer questions carefully. Even if you're happy to take your consultant's advice, it's still important that you have the opportunity to take part in any decisions. You will have more confidence to do this if you don't feel at a disadvantage.

Having someone with you to give you support when you talk to the doctor can help to boost your confidence, particularly if you have worked out together what you want to know beforehand.

Walk-in clinics, mobile screening units and local breast cancer detection campaigns

Normally you have to be referred to a hospital clinic by your GP for further checks and tests but a few hospitals in the country hold walk-in breast clinics which are open to any woman who wishes to attend. These clinics may teach breast self-examination as well as doing a physical examination and, in some cases, a breast X-ray. There are also a few mobile screening units which offer a similar service.

Your area may be one in which a local study has been conducted into early detection for breast cancer either by inviting women to attend a class in breast self-examination or by inviting women to go for a physical examination and a breast X-ray.

Plans are now under way to introduce a mass screening service for the early detection of breast cancer throughout the British Isles. All women between the ages of 50 and 64 will be invited to have a breast X-ray once very three years. (For more information about this see 'Mammography' in Chapter 9.)

Can I change my doctor?

If you're not happy with your GP, perhaps because she has shrugged off your worries or is not prepared to discuss things with you, you may decide you want to change your doctor. This is a simple procedure. Ask the opinion of friends about their doctors. Once you have chosen a new doctor, check with them that their list is open and that they are prepared to accept you. This is a routine procedure and no explanations are needed. Take your medical card to your existing doctor. He will sign it so that you can register with your new doctor. If you need any further help in finding a doctor, you can apply to the Family Practitioner Committee (they're in the phone book).

Can I choose which hospital?

You may live in a city with several hospitals. If you have a preference about which hospital or which consultant you would like
to go to, discuss this with your GP. If she agrees, your appointment will be made with your preference in mind. Your GP probably knows of most of the local consultants who specialize in
breast disease and which ones are sympathetic, so it is worth
asking.

   If you want to attend a hospital in a different area, it may be
a little more difficult. Many consultants are too busy to take women
from outside their locality but this is not always the case. If you
feel strongly that you wish to attend a particular clinic, discuss
this with your doctor so arrangements can be made. (Your regional
health authority will be able to tell you which hospitals have breast
clinics in your area.)

Can I get a second opinion?

If you are not satisfied with the way you have been treated by
your doctor or in hospital, you may want to get a second opinion. While you have no absolute right to one, most doctors and
consultants recognize that having a second opinion may be important if there is any doubt about a diagnosis or proposed treatment.

   I was most dissatisfied with the consultant's approach which
   was patronizing and insulting. I reported this to my GP and
   the next time I found lumps I asked her to refer me to a
   different hospital.

How to complain

If you feel that you want to make a formal complaint about the
way you have been treated by your doctor or in hospital, contact
your local Community Health Council. This body represents our
interests as patients of the NHS. They will advise you how to make
a complaint and help you with any information you need. Each
health authority in the British Isles has a Community Health
Council attached to it. You'll find them in the phone book. Making a complaint can be a complicated business so it is wise to
seek help. (See page 192 for other useful addresses.)

Things to remember when going to the doctor

First, work out beforehand what you want to discuss when you see your doctor. Ask yourself the following questions:

● Do I want to ask my doctor's opinion of what might be wrong before agreeing to go to see a consultant?

● Would I like to discuss with my doctor what might have caused a particular symptom?

● Do I want to discuss other aspects of my health as well?

● If my doctor suggests that I go to an outpatient clinic, do I have a preference about which hospital and which consultant?

● Do I want my doctor to explain what happens in outpatients?

● Do I want to discuss any fears I have about breast cancer, having an appointment at a hospital, etc.?

Second, it is worthwhile writing down your questions and referring to these if you need to. Your GP should never be too busy to discuss with you what might be wrong and what she thinks should be done in your best interests. If you're not satisfied with

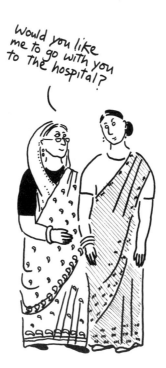

an answer, ask your question again until you receive a satisfac-
tory reply.

Finally, think about taking somebody with you to the doctor's
to give you support and help you find out what you need to know.
If you decide to do this, discuss with them your feelings about
going to the doctor and any worries about your health. In this
way they will be in a better position to give you any support you
need.

Things to remember when preparing for an outpatient appointment

Most of the suggestions made for seeing your doctor apply equally
well when going to see a consultant or registrar in an outpatient
clinic. In addition ask yourself these questions:

● Do I want to take someone with me? Do I want them to be
with me during the interview and the physical examination?

● Do I want to ask about any tests which may be done?

● Do I want to discuss any fears I have about breast cancer with
the doctor in outpatients?

If you decide that you want somebody with you at the interview
and examination, tell the clinic staff. Most hospital doctors don't
mind at all. (Tests you might have are discussed in Chapter 9.)

What to do if you're dissatisfied

If you're not satisfied with what you've been told by your GP, it's
important to tell someone that you're not happy. You could take
one or more of the following steps:

● Go back to your doctor and tell her that you're not happy

● If it's a group practice, see another doctor and explain your
worries

● Go and see another doctor at a local well-woman or family
planning clinic.

If you're not satisfied with what you've been told by the hospital
doctor, you could take the following steps:

● Tell the sister in charge of outpatients that you're worried or
you don't understand

● Ask her how to make an appointment to see your consultant. You are entitled to do this if you want to discuss anything concerning your case

● Ask her if there's another senior doctor you could discuss your worries with

● Go back to your GP and tell her you're unhappy and would like to be referred to another consultant.

Further reading

Anne Dickson, *A Woman in Your Own Right — assertiveness and you* (Quartet Books, 1988).

Stephen Fulder, *How to Survive Medical Treatment — a holistic approach to the risks and side-effects of orthodox medicine* (Century Paperbacks, 1987).

Comments, suggestions and complaints about your stay in hospital, produced by the DHSS.

Patients' Rights: A summary of your rights and responsibilities in the NHS, produced by the National Consumer Council and the Association of Community Health Councils for England and Wales.

CHAPTER NINE
Screening and hospital tests

This chapter discusses the introduction of mass screening for breast cancer in the British Isles and explains its importance in detecting breast cancer. It also looks at different hospital tests which you may undergo if you are referred to hospital as a result of screening or by your GP. It describes the advantages and disadvantages of different tests.

Knowing what's happening when we have a hospital test and understanding what it's for, can help to give us the confidence to voice any queries we might have. The chapter ends by listing some points to consider before agreeing to have a hospital test.

The idea of a hospital test makes most women feel anxious so it's important to remember that the great majority of tests find no evidence of cancer.

Screening

Screening for breast cancer, using physical examination and mammography detects cancers earlier. There is now evidence that early treatment reduces the number of women dying from the disease. Two important studies of mass screening, one in the United States and the other in Sweden, suggest that screening can reduce up to 30 per cent of deaths from breast cancer in women between the ages of 50 and 65. The same evidence of a reduction in deaths through mass screening has not been found for premenopausal women and for women over the age of 65. This may be because mammograms are less reliable in detecting cancer in younger women (see below) and women over 65 have been found less reliable in responding to invitations for screening.

A study by Professor Sir Patrick Forrest has recommended the introduction of mass screening in Britain. The aim is to establish a breast screening centre in every regional health authority in the British Isles. More will be established later as trained staff and cash become available. Screening is extremely costly because of the equipment needed and the intensive training programme required to provide staff for each centre. Because it is so costly, it will be limited to the age group where a definite benefit has been found. Women will be invited once every three years to come to a breast screening centre. Letters will be sent in a similar way to screening for cervical cancer. These centres will be open to any woman who wishes to be screened but because of the doubtful benefits to younger women it is suggested that only those who have a history of breast problems or who are in a risk group (see Chapter 5) should have regular mammograms.

To begin with many women will be referred to hospital after screening but this will not be because of a sudden rise in breast cancer. It will simply reflect the lack of experience in screening staff as centres are established. So it's important not to worry too much if you are referred for a hospital test after screening. Try to remind yourself that up to 90 per cent of those women referred will *not* have cancer.

Critics of mass screening Critics argue that screening can lead to 'over-treatment' of precancerous lumps and non-invasive cancers which may never develop into invasive cancer. They argue that some women will have unnecessary worry or even undergo unnecessary operations as a result.

If you're invited We each need to decide for ourselves if we wish to be screened for breast cancer. Early detection gives us greater choice in how we are treated and increases the chances of a full recovery if we are found to have breast cancer. If you are anxious about having a regular mammogram, remember that most mammograms show no evidence of cancer and the majority of those which appear to show suspicious changes, turn out to be nothing to worry about on further investigation.

Breast x-rays or mammography

A screen test will consist of a breast examination and a breast X-ray. In most cases this will be a mammogram but occasionally ultrasound will be used. A mammogram can pick up small cancers and other abnormalities which aren't yet noticeable to you or your consultant. It's because of this that it will be used in mass screening for breast cancer.

When you go for a mammogram, each breast, in turn, is sandwiched between two X-ray plates. Some women who have tender or painful breasts find this procedure difficult because the breast needs to be firmly held between the plates to get a good image. It's worth telling the radiographer who does the X-ray if you have painful breasts. Some women find this X-ray embarrassing and dehumanizing. If you do, remember you are not alone.

In many hospitals, mammograms are used before any biopsy is performed. The mammogram will show what sort of lump is present (a cyst, a fibroadenoma, a cancer, etc.) and the biopsy will confirm it.

Opinions vary on how accurate mammograms are. Some studies report that mammograms give wrong results in up to 30 per cent of cases. It has been found that mammography is more successful after the menopause. This may be because women who are still having periods tend to have dense breasts which can change considerably in the monthly cycle. Mammograms also carry a small risk of damaging healthy cells (see 'High energy radiation' in Chapter 5). Although this risk is small, it is generally agreed that repeated mammograms are inadvisable in younger women unless they are in one of the categories where there is an increased risk of breast cancer. Then doctors argue that the benefits outweigh any possible risk.

Ultrasound

Ultrasound uses sound waves to create an image of internal organs. The sound waves bounce back different signals (like echoes) depending on the density of the tissue. Some women come across ultrasound during pregnancy where it is used for signs of abnormality in the foetus.

It is particularly useful in looking at very dense breasts. It is accurate with palpable lumps but is unreliable in detecting very small lumps which can't yet be felt. It can also be used to monitor non-cancerous lumps without the hazard of repeated X-rays. Ultrasound is a painless technique which seems to have no harmful side-effects although little is known about its long term use.

Later tests

Mammograms and ultrasound can only suggest something suspicious. To make an accurate diagnosis it is necessary to take a small sample of breast tissue and look at it under a microscope. There is a number of ways that this can be done.

Aspiration cytology: looking at breast cells under a microscope

The study of cells is called cytology.

Breast cells can be removed from the breast using a fine needle on a syringe (similar to an injection needle). This is a simple out-patient procedure which needs no anaesthetic. A consultant will find the lump (or lumpy area) and then hold it securely between the fingers while he inserts the needle into it at a number of different angles. The whole procedure takes about two minutes. Most women feel no pain or discomfort but there may be some bruising afterwards.

> It was the most reassuring and pleasant bit of medicine I've experienced because it was done so quickly and was surprisingly painless. It felt like an injection for a tooth.

If the lump is a cyst it is easily aspirated, and the lump disappears. The fluid aspirated from a cyst may be sent for investigation but this depends on the hospital. Other breast tissue drawn into the syringe is placed on a slide and sent to the laboratory to be checked. Although the results come back within hours, they are normally sent to your doctor or given to you at a later hospital appointment.

It is usual to double-check all non-cancerous results by doing a biopsy in case cancer cells have been missed in this small tissue sample.

Not all hospitals offer aspiration cytology because the technique requires particular skill and experience to obtain a good sample. Many consultants prefer to use a biopsy since in most cases any aspirated lump which isn't obviously a cyst will need further investigation.

Sometimes it's not necessary to use a needle and syringe to test breast fluids. For example, a nipple discharge or an abscess wound can be examined for infection or cell abnormalities by taking a swab.

Biopsy: looking at breast tissue under a microscope

The aim of a biopsy is to provide detailed information about a section of breast tissue containing thousands of cells. Biopsies give the consultant far more information than aspiration cytology. The different methods of biopsy are described in more detail below.

Tru-cut and drill needle biopsies If the lump seems too solid for fine needle aspiration, a needle biopsy may be used. Tru-cut and drill needles are thicker than injection needles and are able to take a small amount of breast tissue from the breast. Because these needles are thicker, a local anaesthetic is given to prevent pain.

The biopsy takes about ten minutes in all, including the time allowed for an injection of local anaesthetic but the time it takes to insert the needle and withdraw a core of tissue is very short — a couple of minutes. The sensation is of someone pushing quite firmly into the breast (about three times). This is normally pain-less but there is often some bruising afterwards.

The tissue is stained with different dyes to highlight the shape and pattern of cells present and so this procedure will take some time to complete. You will either be given a second outpatient appointment a week or so later or the results will be sent on to your own doctor. If the first result shows no cancer cells a further biopsy is often recommended as a double-check.

Excision biopsy Many consultants choose to remove the whole lump under a general anaesthetic. (The word excision means to cut out.) The surgeon will make a small cut along the line of the breast and remove the lump (see diagram on page 119).

This is a minor operation but the general anaesthetic can make some women feel sick and unwell so you may need to stay in hospital for two or three days.

> The first time I had a lump out I went in at 7 a.m. and was finished by 1 p.m. But the second time I was really sick after-wards and had to stay in overnight. I now have matching scars round each nipple, they're very neat!

While the wound is healing, the site of the operation will feel sore, particularly if the weight of the breast drags on the wound. Stitches are removed about a week after your operation. You may have some discomfort until the scar is fully healed. Some women find that the scar remains hard as if the lump is still there.

Like tru-cut and drill biopsies, the lump removed under general anaesthetic will be stained with dyes before being studied under a microscope. The results take a few days to come back from the laboratory so you will either be given an outpatient appointment a week or so later, or the results will be sent on to your doctor.

Excision biopsy is the most accurate form of biopsy.

Frozen section biopsy Because, in a few cases, further treatment may be necessary, some consultants prefer to do a frozen section biopsy. This avoids delay as the breast tissue can be examined while the woman is under a general anaesthetic.

This is the test which gives rise to many of the horror stories in which a woman goes into hospital 'for tests' and wakes up without a breast. The recently revised consent form gives a clearer explanation of the patient's right to information and the doctor's responsibility to explain any treatment to her, so hopefully such horror stories will be a thing of the past. It is very important that before signing the consent form you discuss, with the surgeon, exactly what further measures will be taken if cancer is found.

In this test, a sample of breast tissue is quickly frozen using liquid nitrogen. It is stained, studied under a microscope and the results are sent to the surgeon in the operating theatre. He then continues with more extensive surgery if he thinks it necessary *and* you have given prior consent (see Chapter 12 for details of breast surgery). It is worth remembering that the majority of frozen section biopsies require no further treatment.

Negative results can be double-checked from another sample taken at the same time as the frozen section.

With all the biopsies there are a few borderline cases where the difference between cancerous and non-cancerous cells is difficult to identify. The expertise needed to judge these varies between hospitals so it may be worth asking for a second opinion if your doctor thinks that yours is a borderline case. In general, hospitals which specialize in the treatment of cancer, and breast cancer in particular, have more experienced staff in their laboratories to judge these difficult cases. (This picture will change with the introduction of mass screening centres and improved training for laboratory staff.) It is important to remember that only about 10 per cent of biopsies will be cancerous and a tiny proportion of these will be borderline.

Points to consider when agreeing to have a hospital test

The results of hospital tests are the basis on which any treatment will be decided. As we have seen, no one test is completely superior to the rest, they each have some advantages. What matters is that you have confidence in your choice of test and that you discuss thoroughly any questions, doubts and worries with your GP and consultant before a test and afterwards.

Here are some points to bear in mind:

● Give yourself time to consider which tests you prefer and discuss this with your doctor before you are referred to a hospital consultant

● If your local hospital doesn't do the test you prefer, ask your doctor to refer you to one that does

● If you are dissatisfied with the way a test has been done or the results of a test, you can ask your GP for a second opinion (see Chapter 8)

● If you agree to have a frozen section biopsy discuss with your surgeon what you want to do if cancer is found. Give clear instructions about your choice of treatment

● You could get the opinion of a complementary or alternative health specialist who will help you consider wider issues of your health and any symptoms which seem unrelated to your breasts (see Chapter 10 on how to go about this)

● Only involve yourself in mass screening if you want to

● If you feel yourself becoming over-anxious, seek advice and support from a well-woman clinic, women's health group, or your GP.

Giving yourself time to think

Early treatment of breast cancer is important, but remember that a lump which is found to be cancerous may have developed over several years. Giving yourself time to adjust to your new situation and to work out your choice of treatment after tests are completed won't necessarily harm you, and it may well help you to feel more confident and positive about the treatment you decide upon.

Further reading

Michael Baum, *Breast Cancer: The Facts* (Oxford University Press, 1988), lists the different methods of diagnosis used by modern medicine.

Stephen Fulder, *How To Survive Medical Treatment — a holistic approach to the risks and side-effects of orthodox treatment* (Century Paperbacks, 1987).

The Women's Cancer Control Campaign (see address list page 195), gives information about early screening for breast cancer.

CHAPTER TEN

Seeking help elsewhere

In 1985 over a million British people sought the help of traditional or complementary medicine and many more bought herbal or homoeopathic remedies in health shops and chemists. Also, in the past few years, a number of TV programmes have explored different approaches to health and disease and a wide selection of books on alternative medicine is now available. This chapter looks at some of these health choices and explains how to find out more.

Most alternative practitioners work in private practice. This chapter explains how to find a traditional or complementary practitioner in your area and describes what to expect if you make an appointment to visit one.

Money may be an important question in deciding whether to go to an alternative health professional. This chapter gives an idea of the range of charges and the circumstances in which you may get free treatment or help with charges from the Department of Health and Social Security or private health insurance. Finally some guidelines are suggested on who and what to choose. (A full list of professional bodies representing traditional and complementary medicine can be found on page 198.)

Traditional and complementary health choices

Traditional medicine from China and Japan According to these systems of traditional medicine, all living things are divided into two opposing aspects which are called 'Yin' and 'Yang'. Good health is achieved when yin and yang qualities and organs are in harmony. Illness and disease are caused by an imbalance of these. The characteristics of the body (including feelings and behaviour) are also explained in terms of the natural elements of fire, wood, earth, metal and water. Just as these interact in nature, either in harmony or in opposition, so they are also represented in the different aspects of the human body.

Life and health in the body are believed to stem from a life force or energy called 'Chi'. This vital energy flows around the body through a series of channels or 'meridians'. Any blockage or sluggishness in these channels causes an imbalance which results in ill-health. Different yin organs in the body are matched with yang meridians and vice versa which are in turn linked to the five elements.

Traditional Chinese and Japanese medicine uses a number of therapies which together offer a complete system of health care (surgery is only used as a last resort). These are diet, herbal remedies, heat treatment, massage, acupuncture, acupressure/spot pressing, exercises including breathing and whole-body exercise, meditation and self-healing. All of these are widely practised in the Far East and several, especially acupuncture, are practised in Europe and the United States.

Ayurvedic medicine Ayurvedic medicine is the traditional Hindu medicine and is practised widely in India. In ayurvedic theory, the five senses interact with five basic elements which are the building blocks of all living things (earth, water, fire, air and ether).

Human activity and well-being springs from three inner 'energies' signified by the sun (controlling all biochemical processes), the moon (giving the body form and firmness) and the wind (which corresponds to movement in the body). These inner principles are expressed in character and emotional states as well as physical well-being.

The body is composed of seven different basic tissues. When these are correctly nourished and when the various body channels and water products are correctly balanced, the body is in good health.

Ayurvedic treatments include diet, herbal remedies and drugs, exercise (breathing exercises and whole-body exercises), meditation and self-healing, water therapy and surgery.

There are some practitioners of ayurvedic medicine in Britain, mainly treating people who originate from the Indian subcontinent.

Traditional yoga Traditional yoga is a system of meditation, combining health care with spiritual development. There are several yogic practices including diet, cleansing the body — hygiene, relaxation, breathing exercises, postures or asanas, meditation, contemplation and mystical experience.

Yoga is widely practised in many parts of the world. In Europe and the United States 'hatha' yoga is most popular. This concentrates on breathing and physical postures.

Naturopathy Sometimes called Natural Therapy or Nature Cure in Europe and America, naturopathy uses only natural products in its therapies. These natural remedies cleanse the body of impurities and assist its own self-healing properties. Symptoms are seen as positive signs that the body is trying to correct an imbalance. Treatment is intended to help this process. Naturopathy is practised throughout the world under different names. Treatment includes diet, water therapy, exercise and relaxation. Some naturopaths also use herbal remedies.

Herbalism Herbal medicine is widely practised in most parts of the world. Herbs are used to assist the self-healing properties of the body rather than simply treating symptoms. The aim of herbal medicine is to minimize the development of disease and maximize the body's own ability to heal itself.

Unlike modern medicine's selective use of herb extracts in the production of drugs, all parts of the plant are used in near natural form. Treatments are prepared as tablets or capsules, in liquid form and as ointments or compresses.

Homoeopathy The basis of homoeopathy is that the human body is capable of healing itself because of the presence of a 'vital force' within us. Symptoms are seen as positive signs that our bodies are tackling an illness. The aim of treatment is to use remedies which produce the same symptoms, acting rather like a vaccination to stimulate the body's own healing powers.

Homoeopathy uses pure animal, vegetable and mineral substances. To prepare a remedy the original substance is repeatedly diluted and shaken (succussed). It is thought that this process increases the 'power' or potency of the remedy. It also makes it completely safe as little or nothing of the original substance remains.

Homoeopathy is practised throughout Europe and is also widely used in India. In Britain it is available on the NHS (see further on).

Anthroposophy Anthroposophy is a twentieth century alternative approach to medicine. It emphasizes the spiritual and emotional aspects of humanity. Humans are believed to have four separate qualities or 'bodies'; the physical body of organs and systems; the 'etheric' body of creative forces and energies; the 'astral' body of feeling and emotions; and the 'ego' or human spirit.

These four elements interact and any imbalance results in ill-health.

Anthroposophy has several different approaches to treatment. These include diet, herbal remedies, homoeopathic remedies, conventional drugs, water therapy, massage, movement therapy, art and music therapy and special anthroposophic preparations.

Anthroposophy is mainly practised in Switzerland and Austria. There are a few doctors in Britain who use this approach. Some anthroposophic remedies are used by homoeopaths.

Nutritional medicine It is now well known that some refined foods, artificial additives, colours and preservatives have a harmful effect on our health. It is also recognized that each person has different nutritional needs. Nutritional medicine uses the knowledge of western science to assess the quality of nourishment in our diet at different times in our lives and in different situations. Nutritionists analyse each diet, pointing out any imbalance or deficiency. They are able to advise on a healthy diet and on any supplements of vitamins and minerals which can improve health and help to treat disease.

Alexander Technique Our posture and the way we move is often the result of years of tension, lack of confidence and bad habits. The Alexander Technique is based on the theory that, with practice, we can undo years of poor posture which can not only relieve back pain, shoulder pain and round shoulders but also improve our self-confidence.

A teacher explains through demonstration and exercise new ways in which the individual can learn to stand, sit, move and relax. With practice, these techniques are intended to become effortless and beneficial, both psychologically and physically.

Healing All health workers see themselves as healers but there is a long tradition which recognizes that some people have special healing powers. Often these powers are seen as a religious or spiritual gift but not all healers are religious nor do they require that you believe before they treat you.

Healing can take place with the healer present or at a distance with contact by post or by phone. It can include meditation, prayers and the 'laying-on-of-hands'.

Counselling and psychotherapy

Mental and emotional factors in ill-health have been recognized for thousands of years in traditional medicines, but psychology (the study of mental processes) and psychiatry (the study of personality formation and behaviour disorders) are still relatively young fields in modern science. Modern medicine is becoming more aware of the value of mental and psychological approaches to ill-health but, due to lack of resources, the possibility of such treatment often remains limited to life crises and mental illness. This is not true for those GPs who see counselling and psychotherapy as a central part of their work. The problem arises when more specialized help is required.

There are several kinds of therapy. A counseller takes an active role in advising and supporting the person counselled. A psychotherapist is there to support the person in self-discovery and understanding. Counselling and psychotherapy can include one-to-one contact, group therapy, mental imagery or visualization, relaxation exercises, meditation, breathing and whole-body exercises, art and music therapy and hypnotism.

How to find out more

Traditional and complementary health workers may work in specialist clinics, general clinics or health centres (which offer a number of alternative treatments), as a member of an NHS health practice (although this is unusual) or as individuals, sometimes working from home. There are also a few doctors and nurses who have done some training in a particular area of traditional or complementary medicine and who may offer these in your local surgery, although this is not common.

There are a number of ways to find out what is available in your area:

● Your local Civic Information Service, attached to the local library, may have a list of different practitioners in the area

● The national professional bodies of each type of medicine hold an up-to-date list of all those practising (see page 192)

● Health shops or whole-food shops may carry a list or be able to put you in touch with a particular practitioner

● Chemists who stock herbal and homoeopathic remedies often know of local herbalists and homoeopaths and may know about other practitioners

● Yellow Pages lists some of the more well-known therapies

● Health groups and health education classes sometimes share experiences and information about local practitioners

● Centres for traditional and complementary medicine often produce their own publicity. They may organize 'open days' so that people can find out more

● By word of mouth. A surprising number of people will have some experience or know someone who has been to see an alternative practitioner

● Most traditional and complementary practitioners know what other therapies are available in the area and have no objection to answering your enquiry about these

● Sometimes public meetings or day-schools about alternatives to modern medicine in general, or a particular alternative medicine, are advertised in the local press or library.

Most traditional and complementary practitioners are happy for you to discuss the possibility of treatment before any appointment is made. You may want to know what to expect and you will certainly want to know how much it will cost. Most national bodies will send you information explaining the basic principles of their approach if you ask them.

What to expect when you visit an alternative health specialist

The first visit to a practioner of traditional or complementary medicine is usually the most expensive and takes the longest (usually an hour to an hour and a half). The practitioner will want to map out a history of your health and that of your family. You may be asked about your birth, any childhood illnesses or major diseases, whether you've had an operation, and there may be questions about your reproductive life. Similar questions may be asked about sisters and brothers, parents and even grandparents. (It may be difficult to remember these details so it is helpful to write some notes beforehand.)

You will then be asked about your present state of health. This will range from questions about the effects of work or unemployment, to whether your skin is dry, whether you sleep well at night or feel tired and lacking in energy. You will be asked about your worries and your fears and the major stresses in your life. You will also be asked if you are receiving any conventional treatments.

After this interview is completed, you may be given a thorough physical examination, not only of your breasts but of all the major organs and parts of the body. Only when this interview and examination is complete is there any discussion about what might be wrong and recommendations made about treatment.

Some alternative practitioners may use additional techniques to help their diagnosis. For example, traditional Chinese practitioners believe that a study of the body pulses in the wrist, the neck and the leg arteries can tell them about the state of internal organs. Techniques used by other therapists include the study of the iris in the eyes and the analysis of blood or hair to detect mineral deficiency.

Most traditional and complementary therapists will discuss with you the possibility and, in some cases, the importance of combining an alternative diagnosis with a conventional medical diagnosis. For many women the value of an alternative diagnosis lies in the opportunity it gives us to discuss fully what may be wrong and to consider other aspects of our health needs not covered by modern medicine.

> I've had breast lumps and breast problems for years and I never had a proper explanation until I went to an alternative doctor. I was given a thorough examination of my breasts and my whole body and she explained to me how different types of lumps developed, why my breasts were painful and tender and then worked out a programme of treatment of diet, water therapy and breast exercises, explaining exactly what each was going to do. The treatment has really helped. I combine this with yearly check-ups at the hospital.

After your first appointment others may be suggested on a monthly, three-monthly or six-monthly basis to monitor the value of any treatment undertaken. These may be less expensive and usually take less time (about half an hour to an hour).

Some alternative practitioners are prepared to advise you on health matters at a distance if travel is a problem. This may involve filling in a detailed questionnaire and arranging to have either a written or a telephone consultation. Either way you will have to pay some kind of fee.

How to choose which practitioner

Decide which therapy interests you and contact the appropriate national professional body for a list of qualified practitioners in your area. You may know someone who's been to an alternative practitioner. A personal recommendation is always helpful.

Check with the practitioner that they are properly qualified. Ask them where they trained and what qualification they have.

It is better to travel to an experienced and qualified practitioner in another area than go to someone local whose knowledge and experience is limited to a correspondence or six-month training course.

Do you tell your doctor or consultant?

Many doctors are hostile to traditional and complementary medicine. You will have to assess whether you want them to know if you go to see an alternative practitioner. It is probably best to sound out your doctor before declaring yourself. Any qualified practitioner will tell you if you need to inform your doctor about treatment you are receiving.

The problem of finance and what to do about it

The problem of money stops many people from seeking the advice of alternative practitioners in private practice. A first consultation can cost £15 to £30 with follow-up treatment at £10 to £20. For many people on low incomes, paying for a consultation is a luxury they cannot afford. Only if modern medicine fails to cure recurrent ill-health do most people turn, in desperation, to alternative help.

Free services The department of Health and Social Security rarely agrees to pay for alternative treatments because most traditional and complementary practitioners are not registered under the various medical acts. There are, however, some important exceptions.

Homoeopaths are permitted to practise under the NHS provided they are qualified doctors. There are a number of homoeopathic hospitals and clinics (see address list on page 192) and a few doctors in general practice offer both modern and homoeopathic therapies. Also, an increasing number of health professionals and doctors are training in acupuncture. There are individual cases where people have been referred by their doctor or consultant to an osteopath or chiropractor (similar to an osteopath). Some herbal remedies can be obtained on prescription.

Private medical insurance takes a similar position to the DHSS, only reimbursing claims for treatment from registered medical practitioners. Nevertheless, there are cases where the rules have been waived and fees for a number of treatments have been paid. If you have a private policy it is worth checking in what circumstances, if any, you can claim for alternative treatments.

Reduced charges Many traditional and complementary practitioners are well aware of differences in the incomes of the people they see and operate a sliding scale of charges to 'help' unemployed and low paid patients. This is something you should discuss before the consultation. If you can't afford to see a traditional or complementary practitioner, there is still the helpful advice of herbal and homoeopathic chemists.

Widening our choices

Traditional and complementary therapies can be helpful in a number of different ways. We can use their whole-person approach and their 'gentle' remedies to improve the quality of our health and to help prevent disease. If we become ill, we can combine traditional and complementary treatments with modern medicine to make sure that all aspects of our health are looked after. And we can use them to counter some of the harmful side-effects of modern medicine. Finally we can choose traditional and complementary treatments instead of modern treatments if we have more confidence in them. Having that choice and having the confidence to act on it will provide the best possible conditions for recovery and good health.

Further reading

Victor Batt, *Anthroposophical Medicine — an extension of the art of healing* (Rudolph Steiner Press, 1982).

Penny Brohn, *The Bristol Programme — an introduction to the holistic therapies practised by the Bristol Cancer Help Centre* (Century Paperbacks, 1987).

Dr. Stephen Davies and Dr. Alan Stewart, *Nutritional Medicine — the drug free guide to better family health* (Pan Books, 1987).

Birgit Heyn, *Ayurvedic medicine* (Thorsons, 1987).

Brian Ingliss and Ruth West, *The Alternative Health Guide* (Michael Joseph, 1988).

Dr. Felix Mann, *Acupuncture — how it works and how it is used today* (Pan Books, 1985).

Chee Soo, *The Taoist Ways of Healing* (Aquarian Press, 1986).

Dr. Andrew Stanway, *Alternative Medicine — A guide to natural therapies* (Penguin, 1986).

George Vithoulkas, *Homeopathy — medicine of the new man* (Thorsons, 1979).

CHAPTER ELEVEN
Different treatments for breast problems and non-cancerous breast disease

As we saw in Chapter 3, non-cancerous breast disorders can take many different forms. This chapter looks at different treatments to these problems. Modern medicine uses a number of approaches including vitamins, changes in diet, drugs, antibiotics, drainage of fluids and surgery. X-rays and ultrasound may also be used to monitor different conditions.

There are also a number of alternative ways to treat breast problems and non-cancerous breast disease. These include diet, vitamin and mineral supplements, herbal preparations, water therapy, breast exercises and relaxation exercises to relieve stress. Traditional and complementary practitioners may also have recommendations about herbal or homoeopathic remedies, acupuncture and acupressure, but these are not standard treatments. They will usually be tailored to the individual needs of each woman.

Not all breast problems are 'physical' in nature. Some women feel deeply unhappy about the size and appearance of their breasts and this can undermine their confidence and dominate their lives. The chapter looks at this problem and suggests ways of treating it.

Treatments for premenstrual swelling and tenderness

Many women experience some swelling and tenderness leading up to a period. Sometimes it can disrupt our social lives and make us feel depressed and ill. Most women find they have to experiment with different approaches before they find out what works for them. Hopefully these suggestions will give you some good ideas.

Diet Some foods seem to affect breast tenderness and swelling directly, for example coffee. Your doctor may suggest you cut out coffee and possibly tea, alcohol and smoking as well. Traditional and complementary therapists are likely to go much further in advising you to change your diet. This is because a healthy diet is seen as an essential first step in treating ill-health. Different therapists may recommend different diets but they are likely to share the same basic advice:

● Cut down on and try to cut out tea, coffee, salt, alcohol, white flour products, white sugar products, tinned foods and any foods which have additives and preservatives in them

● Reduce intake of fats, particularly animal fats and dairy produce

● Cut down on and try to cut out red meat which may have additives like growth hormones in it

● Eat fish, poultry, whole-grains and pulses (peas, beans, lentils, etc.) for protein

● Increase the amount of fibre in your diet, particularly vegetables and fruit

● If you're overweight, try to lose some weight.

If you want to change your diet, it is important not to set yourself impossible goals. The point is to work out a diet which you can stick to and which improves your health and your own sense of well-being.

> For years, I had a lot of premenstrual problems and very painful breasts. Now, I keep a generally healthy diet throughout the month but about a week before my period, I cut out protein, cheese and I go off alcohol completely and switch to eating fruit and veg, almost entirely. I find it works quite effectively. And I drink parsley tea which is disgusting but brilliant.

Vitamin and mineral supplements Your doctor may suggest you try vitamin B_6 (called pyridoxine). Some women find this very useful but others find it makes no difference. Other supplements recommended by nutritionists which you may wish to discuss with your doctor are listed below:

Multivitamin supplement which includes vitamins, minerals and trace elements. Drs Stephen Davies and Alan Stewart recommend the multivitamin Optivite — see reading list at the end of the chapter

Evening Primrose Oil (500 mg capsules). Take 4 — 8 a day for two weeks before your period. It works best with a multivitamin and trace element supplement

Vitamin E (300 — 500 International Units per day) has been found to be helpful for breast tenderness and swelling

Magnesium supplement (200 — 300 mg per day). This is best taken with multivitamin supplement.

(See *Nutritional Medicine* recommended in the reading list.)

Vitamins are expensive so investigate the possibility of getting them on prescription (see page 151). It is worth noting that some doctors are unwilling to prescribe vitamins and minerals in this way.

Diuretics Diuretics are drugs which help to relieve fluid retention in the body by stimulating the kidneys to release more fluids in the form of urine.

Several natural diuretics help to reduce fluid retention. In particular, naturopaths recommend cucumber, parsley, grapefruit, potatoes, apples and white grapes.

There are also herbal diuretics which can be obtained from herbal chemists, health shops and some larger chemists. Some brand names are Waterfall, Health and Heather Diuretic, Couch Grass capsules and Potters Diuretabs. (Bear in mind that a trained herbalist or homoeopath will prescribe a remedy based on a full diagnosis but this is not available over the counter.)

You can also buy a mild chemical diuretic in most chemists, for example Aquaban, but anything stronger will need a prescription. There are a number of chemical diuretic drugs which your doctor may suggest. All of them have some potential side-effects, but these are rare, particularly if taken for short periods of time.

Chemical diuretic drugs

Diuretic	Possible side-effects
Bendrofluazide and other thiazides	Rashes, temporary impotence, long term use may lead to gout or diabetes
Moduretic	Headache, weakness, dizziness, cramps, drowsiness in some people
Frusemide (Lasix)	Nausea, gastric upset, weakness in some people

Reading about the side-effects of drugs can cause anxiety which may result in the expected side-effect, so it's important to remember that few women have side-effects from diuretic drugs and any unpleasant symptoms will stop once treatment ceases.

Water therapy Some traditional and complementary practitioners recommend water therapy for premenstrual breast tenderness and swelling. This involves spraying your breasts with cold water once or twice a day on a regular basis. The aim of this is to stimulate the blood supply and 'tone-up' breast tissue. Some practitioners argue that regular water therapy in adult life can help to prevent many breast disorders from developing.

Breast exercises and other forms of exercise Breast exercises, sometimes called pectoral exercises, have also been found to be useful and can be combined with water sprays, morning and night (see page 53).

Exercise can help to ease tension which sometimes increases the symptoms of breast pain and swelling. Regular exercise, like swimming once a week, can be helpful (see suggestions on page 53). Yoga exercises are also useful for learning how to relax and improve your posture or you may prefer to use the Alexander Technique or Chinese exercises if instruction is available in your area.

> I've been using diet, breast exercises and spraying my breasts off and on for the last five years. Whenever my breasts get really achy and painful, I start doing the exercises and water sprays every night and morning and it works. I don't know why. I sometimes think it's because I'm doing something positive for myself and my breasts appreciate it.

Sore nipples and breast infections during breastfeeding

Problems in breastfeeding can often be prevented by careful preparation before the birth and in the early days of breastfeeding, and by a healthy diet and enough rest. For busy mothers this is harder than it sounds!

If you prefer not to breastfeed you may experience some discomfort for a few days while the milk dries up in your breasts. If you start to breastfeed, and then stop, the process is more complicated: you may experience painful, swollen breasts and may need an injection to stop the milk flow. In this situation, reducing fluid intake can help. If your baby is too ill to be put to the breast or you are in need of treatment, yourself, you can express the milk from your breasts in readiness and, if necessary, store it for use while you or the baby are unable to breastfeed. A number of mechanical expressers are available. Your doctor will be able to advise you on which type will suit your needs best.

If your nipples become sore or cracked when you breastfeed, your GP can prescribe a mild ointment, such as Kamillosan, to lubricate them. Or you can buy a mild oil like wheat germ oil, or calendula (a homoeopathic ointment) from most herbalists and health food shops. It's important to try to keep breastfeeding even though your breasts are sore so that they don't become engorged, which will increase the likelihood of infection. If the nipple is very sore, you could gently express some of the milk in that breast and then give the nipple a rest so that it has a chance to heal. It won't harm the baby if you only feed from one breast for a few days.

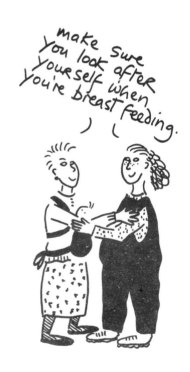

Mastitis

If one breast becomes sore and tender with the beginnings of infection (mastitis) you may feel feverish and have symptoms of 'flu' (often this is due to inflammation rather than infection). Try to continue breastfeeding. Draining the breast helps to clear the infection and it doesn't harm the baby. Try feeding more frequently so that the baby is less hungry and energetic when it feeds. This ensures that the infected milk ducts are being regularly drained. By doing this you can help to stop an infection before it gets hold.

In the early stages of a breast infection, some midwives suggest soaking or bathing the breast regularly in hot water. Some women prefer ice and cold compresses instead. Midwives advise as much complete rest as possible.

If the infection doesn't go, your doctor may suggest a course of antibiotics. Antibiotics are effective in tackling invading bacteria. The problem is, they also occasionally have side-effects such as digestive problems, tiredness and headaches and some people have an allergic reaction to certain kinds. Antibiotics also tend to be over-prescribed.

While you're taking a course of antibiotics, try to keep up your nourishing diet and periods of rest, as well as bathing your breasts with hot water, or ice if you prefer, because these will all help speed up your recovery.

Here are some ideas which may help if you're worried about taking antibiotics:

● Eat live yogurt which helps if antibiotics cause digestive problems

● Take extra vitamins, particularly vitamin C

● Note any allergic reaction and tell your doctor as early as possible

● Continue to treat yourself carefully for at least ten days after the infection so that your body can fully recover.

Most doctors would advise you to continue breastfeeding while you are taking antibiotics so that the milk ducts are regularly drained. This isn't an ideal situation for a young baby, but doctors feel that breastfeeding helps to clear the infection quickly and is in the best long-term interests of the infant. Most babies appear not to be seriously affected by antibiotics in breast milk, but keep an eye out for unusual rashes or colicky behaviour. If you don't want to feed your baby while you're taking antibiotics, express the milk from your breasts until the infection has cleared up and then continue breastfeeding. Whichever you choose, it is important to drain the breast frequently because this will help to clear the infection.

Traditional and complementary practitioners are wary of antibiotics, arguing that they suppress any symptoms and prevent the body from healing itself. They prefer to emphasize the healing measures of diet, rest and water therapy. They may also recommend herbal and homoeopathic remedies in place of antibiotics. Whichever choice you make, it's best to seek help early if you think you're getting a breast infection.

Breast abscess

Occasionally an abscess can develop which may require minor surgery, under local or general anaesthetic, to remove the pus and install a drain. This complication is rare and usually the result of poor health and poor treatment. A breast abscess may take several weeks to heal. Diet and rest will help and some women find that herbal or homoeopathic remedies can speed up the healing process as well.

Modern treatments of non-cancerous breast disease

Some non-cancerous conditions are easily identified. But many others share the same symptoms as breast cancer, so a doctor's first concern is to rule out this small possibility (see 'Screening and hospital tests', page 76). The aim of most of these tests is to check for cancer rather than to cure the non-cancerous condition.

Surgery Ducts which contain a papilloma or duct ectasia may be surgically removed by cutting around the areola and lifting the skin to reveal the underlying ducts.

Occasionally duct ectasia becomes infected producing a recurring abscess condition which may require surgery. In very rare circumstances, the infected area is both widespread and recurring and so unpleasant for the woman concerned that doctors may suggest a subcutaneous mastectomy (see page 109).

Hormone-related drugs Breast pain is a symptom of several non-cancerous conditions and is extremely common. It is thought to be caused by an imbalance in hormone levels of oestrogen, progesterone and prolactin. Medical science has developed several hormone-related drugs which attempt to correct these imbalances. All these drugs may have side-effects in a few women.

Hormonal drugs

Hormonal drug	Possible side-effects
Progesterone (pessary injection, or tablets) and *Dydrogesterone* (both these drugs alter the balance between oestrogen and progesterone)	Weight gain, acne, gastric disturbance, water retention, breast discomfort, changes in sex drive, irregular periods
Bromocriptine (restrains the production of prolactin)	Nausea, vomiting, constipation, headache, dizziness, drowsiness, hypotension (low blood pressure)
Danazol (acts on the pituitary, reducing hormones which stimulate the ovary to secrete oestrogen and progesterone)	Nausea, dizziness, rashes, backache, flushing, acne, oily skin, vertigo, fluid retention and increased body hair; low doses of Danazol reduce these side-effects considerably

Treatment works for some women but not for others. In the same way, some women will have few side-effects while others will feel quite unwell. Any side-effects should stop once treatment has ceased. Hormonal drugs are only prescribed if a woman is experiencing considerable and prolonged pain in her breasts. Before agreeing to these drugs, you may wish to see an alternative practitioner (see below and chapter 10).

In a very few cases, constant pain or discomfort doesn't respond to the drugs presently available. If a woman's quality of life is severely affected by pain, doctors may suggest surgery to remove the breast. This is extremely rare and only undertaken if it is the woman's wish (see subcutaneous mastectomy page 109).

Traditional and complementary treatments for non-cancerous breast disease

The remedies described earlier in this chapter — diet, vitamin supplements, water therapy, breast exercises, whole-body exercise and herbal and homoeopathic preparations — can be helpful for breast lumps and other symptoms. You should try to see an experienced and qualified alternative practitioner to work out which remedies will help your particular problem. It may mean setting yourself a target to use the treatments for three months to see if they work for you. This can be done while you remain under the eye of a hospital consultant or you can decide to give yourself a break from hospitals and tests.

For women with non-cancerous breast disease who do not want drugs or continued hospital treatment, traditional and complementary medicine can provide an alternative avenue to good health. At the same time, it is important that any new symptoms are properly investigated by your GP or a consultant.

Feeling unhappy about our breasts

Psychological support

Western preoccupation with the female form, and women's breasts in particular, has some effect on most women. A few women become deeply preoccupied with the appearance of their breasts. They may seem too large, too small or they may have changed shape with increasing age. If negative feelings about your breasts and your body-image are sapping your confidence and making life miserable or even making you physically ill (some women have chronic backache, slumped shoulders, difficulty in breathing), it is important to find some sympathetic help. You may get that support from a women's group although not every woman has the confidence or the opportunity to go along regularly to a local group.

Another possibility is to ask your doctor to put you in touch with a counsellor or psychotherapist who can help you work through your feelings about your breasts. This may be available on the NHS, or through a charitable/voluntary organization or a private practitioner. You may find that you need to see someone on a regular basis for a year or more — however long it takes to regain your confidence and feel positive about your body. With support and understanding most women can overcome these disabling feelings about themselves.

Cosmetic surgery

There is also the choice of cosmetic surgery to alter the appearance of our breasts. This drastic step is only available on the NHS if it is established that a woman is severely affected by anxiety so that her quality of life is undermined. Most women who have cosmetic surgery pay to have it done privately.

Breast enlargement Breasts can be made larger by inserting a silicon implant or prosthesis into the breast. This is usually done by making a cut beneath the breast and inserting the silicon prosthesis from below before stitching the wound up.

Alternatively a cut can be made around the areola and nipple and an inflatable prosthesis can be inserted beneath the nipple area. Once the operation has healed, the breast can function as before although some women lose some feeling in their nipples. Women who have had their breasts enlarged are usually able to breastfeed.

Breast enlargment can have complications. Sometimes the silicon implant becomes gradually enfolded in fibrous tissue and this can harden the area so that the breast shape becomes distorted. This can be painful. In most cases, the implant will be removed and a new one inserted before such complications arise.

Reduction in breast size There are several variations to this operation. One method moves the nipple and areola and places it higher on the breast, at the same time removing an area of breast tissue below. This may affect sensation in the nipple. A second method cuts away some breast tissue and folds the remainder in on itself beneath the nipple area.

If you decide you need cosmetic surgery, it is a good idea to ask your surgeon about possible complications and drawbacks before you make any decision to go ahead.

Making choices

Breast problems and non-cancerous breast conditions can be helped by improving the quality of our diet and overall health. In many cases these breast disorders can be successfully treated either by modern medicine or by traditional and complementary medicine.

You will need to find out for yourself which treatment suits you best. More and more women are finding that their choices include traditional and complementary therapies. In most cases, these treatments are combined with monitoring breast changes through mammography or biopsy in the normal way. Whatever the problem, it's worth finding out about *all* the choices that are available. You may need to look beyond the confines of modern medicine to find a whole-woman approach to your health care.

Further reading

Dorothy Brewster, *You Can Breastfeed Your Baby Too... Even in Special situations* (Rodale Press, 1979).

Dr. Stephen Davies and Dr. Alan Stewart, *Nutritional Medicine* (Pan Books, 1987).

Patrick Holford, *The Whole Health Manual* (Thorsons, 1983).

Maire Messenger Davies, *The Breastfeeding Book* Century Paperbacks (1982).

Angela Phillips and Jill Rakusen, *Our Bodies—Our Selves: A health book by and for women* (Penguin Books, 1987).

CHAPTER TWELVE

Modern treatments for primary breast cancer

Finding out you have breast cancer

No woman can predict how she will feel when she is told she has breast cancer. Some women are too stunned to take the information in, others feel angry and bitter. Some women have the love and support of those near to them to hear this unwelcome news but others may face the news alone.

When you are first told your diagnosis you may feel too upset to take in fully what is wrong and what choices of treatment are available. Some consultants leave their patients for a few minutes so that they can collect their thoughts before returning to discuss treatment with them. Don't be afraid to ask your consultant to leave you for a few minutes if this is what you would like. In hospitals where there is a breast care nurse, she may attend the interview and try to give you some support after the consultant has gone. Find out if your hospital has a breast care nurse and ask to see her if you'd like to.

Sorting out your thoughts may take some time and while you will be encouraged to have surgery as soon as possible, it's important to give yourself time to find out what you want to know and how you want to be treated. This may mean a second appointment to see the consultant. You are entitled to ask for this and most consultants are very happy to go over things again so you are confident about your decisions.

The aim of the next part of this book is to spell out what is involved in different treatments for breast cancer so that you are in a better position to feel confident and informed about how you wish to be treated. Chapters 12 to 16 look at modern treatments for breast cancer and Chapter 17 looks at traditional and complementary choices you may wish to follow. Different women

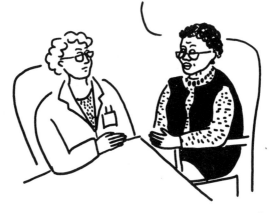

I want to be clear in my own mind before I agree to any treatment.

will make very different decisions about treatment, including asking their consultant to make all decisions for them. What is important is that you are confident in the choices you have made. Experience shows that confidence helps the process of recovery and adjustment to a new period of your life.

This chapter looks at modern methods of treating primary breast cancer. A primary breast cancer is a cancer which has started in breast tissue and where there is no sign of cancer spread. (With early detection and greater awareness among women, this is the most common form of breast cancer.) As we have seen, there are a number of different breast cancers, some slow-growing, others not. Some remain in the breast and some may spread to other parts of the body.

For most women the first line of treatment for primary breast cancer is surgery, combined in some cases with radiotherapy. This chapter describes different forms of surgery. It explains how radiotherapy works and what side-effects it has. It also looks at differences of opinion within the medical profession about treating primary breast cancer. The chapter ends by stressing the importance of our participation in decisions about treatment.

Elderly women and women with advanced cancers may not have surgery. Instead they may be offered some form of drug therapy (see Chapters 16 and 19).

Different forms of surgery

The technical term used for the surgical removal of the breast is mastectomy. The aim of mastectomy operations has been to remove all trace of cancer cells from the breast and surrounding tissue. Other forms of surgery remove a part of the breast (partial mastectomy) or an area immediately surrounding the cancer (lumpectomy).

Simple mastectomy with or without lymph node sample

This operation removes the breast tissue. Some surgeons may also take a sample of lymph nodes in the armpit to check if any cancer cells are present. If the cancer is on the inner side of the breast, some lymph nodes beneath the breast bone may be looked at for the same reason. How many lymph nodes are removed will depend on the surgeon.

Partial mastectomy with or without lymph node sample

This operation, sometimes called 'quadrectomy' or 'segmentectomy' removes a wedge-like slice of the breast. If this is far from the axillary tail of the breast where lymph nodes can be found, a separate incision may be made to remove a sample of lymph nodes. While a partial mastectomy leaves most of the breast intact, it can change the shape of the breast and may include removal of the nipple.

Lumpectomy with or without axillary node sample

This operation is the same as excision biopsy. The lump is removed with some surrounding breast tissue. If the lump is near the axillary tail, a sample of lymph nodes can be removed at the same time. Otherwise another incision may be made.

In most cases a partial mastectomy or a lumpectomy will be followed by a course of radiotherapy.

There are two further forms of mastectomy which were the standard treatment for breast cancer for many years but which now are performed less often.

Modified radical mastectomy

This operation removes the breast tissue and all the lymph nodes in the armpit (the technical term for removing all lymph nodes is 'dissection of the lymph nodes')

Radical mastectomy

For years surgeons thought the only way of ensuring that all trace of cancer cells had been removed was to remove not only the breast but also the underlying chest muscle and the lymph nodes in the armpit. This meant taking a large area of body tissue in a woman's chest and shoulder. (A 'super-radical mastectomy' removes all the interior lymph nodes under the breast bone as well.)

As more has become known about breast cancer and as smaller cancers are treated earlier, the routine use of radical mastectomy and super-radical mastectomy has declined in favour of less severe measures.

Several studies comparing radical surgery with simple mastectomy, or with partial mastectomy and lumpectomy followed by radiotherapy, have shown a similar rate of success in treating primary breast cancer. Doctors have also become far more aware of the distress experienced in losing a breast and now recognize that many women will want to keep their breasts if possible.

The side-effects of surgery

Most of the side-effects of surgery pass with time as the wound heals and as the woman recovers from the effects of the anaesthetic.

Most women will find their scars fade well but not all women are as lucky. If you have a tendency to scar badly or if you have a tendency to develop keloid scarring (this increases the scar tissue and is more common in black women), you may want to discuss this with your surgeon. It may also affect your choice of surgery (see Chapter 13 for more information about side-effects).

Radiotherapy: what it does and how it is used

Treatment using ionizing radiation (called radiation therapy or radiotherapy) is a second form of treatment for primary breast cancer. Radiation works by sending ionizing rays into the breast.

These rays interfere with the DNA (the genetic blueprint in each cell). Cells have an ability to correct such interference, given time. Healthy cells in the breasts have long periods of rest between each cell division and so the great majority of them are able to correct any interference from ionizing rays. But if cells are dividing rapidly, this corrective mechanism hasn't time to work. Cancer cells tend to divide more rapidly than healthy cells, and so remain damaged when they come to duplicate themselves. The result is that new cancer cells are so badly damaged they stop functioning and die.

Radiotherapy is started as soon as any surgery has healed. It can be given weekly, twice weekly and in some instances daily. Treatment lasts a few minutes each time and may spread over several weeks. (See 'Radiotherapy — what to expect', page 127.)

The side-effects of radiotherapy

Radiotherapy has a number of possible side-effects. These affect some women more than others.

● Many women complain of tiredness and depression both during radiotherapy and for some time afterwards

● The skin of the immediate area may become red and sore rather like sunburn and it may become dry and flaky. (Fair skinned women, particularly those with red hair, are likely to be most sensitive to these side-effects.) This soreness may last some weeks after treatment has finished

● The skin area may change colour (either lighter or darker). This discoloration gradually disappears after treatment but occasionally it may remain permanently

● The skin may 'weep' if it is rubbed or accidentally broken (this will eventually heal after treatment has finished)

● The hair in the armpit will fall out but this will soon grow again once treatment has finished. No other body hair is affected

● There may be thickening or fibrosis at the site of the radiotherapy. This thickening can make your breast feel different and less sensitive to touch. Occasionally fibrosis of lung tissue can occur. This can lead to shortness of breath and other lung complaints

● If the armpit is irradiated, fluid retention (lymphoedema) is possible. This may cause discomfort and swelling in the arm

● The immune system is affected by radiation and it may take some years to recover fully

- With any course of radiation therapy, there is a slightly increased chance of secondary cancers developing later in life

- Some women complain of pain following radiotherapy.

Most side-effects should go within a few weeks. Those side-effects which in some women are permanent have to be weighed against the increased likelihood of local recurrence if the consultant says there is evidence of local spread or if a partial mastectomy or lumpectomy is performed. Some women will prefer to have a mastectomy *without* radiotherapy rather than a lumpectomy *with* radiotherapy. These are points you may want to raise with your doctor, your consultant or the breast care nurse when you are in hospital. (Chapter 14 looks at ways in which the side-effects of radiotherapy can be reduced.)

Breast reconstruction

In recent years some surgeons have turned their attention to breast reconstruction after surgery. The aim of reconstruction is to create a breast form with a cleavage which will appear natural in almost all situations except when you are naked. Of course it doesn't look exactly like the original but it does make mastectomy easier to live with for many women.

Breast reconstruction at the time of mastectomy
This can be performed at the same time as a simple or modified radical mastectomy. The surgeon places a silicon implant underneath the large chest muscle. This provides a rounded shape or 'breast mound' on which a nipple and areola can be constructed later. This can be done by grafting skin from the inside of the thigh onto the breast mound. An alternative is to use a detachable silicon nipple.

Breast reconstruction after mastectomy
This is either offered several months later so that a woman has time to consider if she wants a reconstructed breast or it is offered to women who had a mastectomy several years ago before breast reconstruction was widely available.

   How the reconstruction is done depends on the original mastectomy. Different methods can be used depending on how much breast muscle has been removed and the quality of the skin covering the site of the operation. If the underlying breast muscles remain intact, a silicon implant can be placed beneath the large breast muscle. If there isn't enough skin cover at the mastectomy site, skin can be gently expanded using an inflatable implant or it can sometimes be grafted from beneath the breast area. A silicon implant can then be inserted at a later date. If some of the breast muscle has been removed in surgery, muscle from behind the arm or from the abdomen may be used. This involves major surgery before an implant can be inserted beneath the new muscle.

Subcutaneous mastectomy

This involves removing all the underlying breast tissue and leaving the skin and nipple intact. A silicon implant is then placed in the breast area either at the same time or at a later date. If it's done later, the skin over the breast is first gently expanded using an inflatable silicon implant before a permanent implant is put into position.

Subcutaneous mastectomy is more likely to be used in noncancerous breast disease. It will only be offered to women with breast cancer if the surgeon is satisfied that there is no likelihood of recurrence of cancer in the skin and nipple.

Breast reconstruction does have some limitations. It is really only possible in women with small breasts. It may involve more than one operation to create the possibility of an implanted breast form. It *may* mean an operation to the second breast so that both breasts are the same size. Any changes in breast shape due to increasing age or weight will also tend to create a lopsided figure. If the implant becomes enfolded in fibrous tissue, there is the possibility of contraction (see 'Breast enlargement' page 100).

It is important to discuss these problems before you agree to have reconstruction surgery. Your surgeon will have photographs which you can look at and the Breast Care and Mastectomy Association will discuss with you any queries you have and put you in touch with women in your area who have had reconstruction at the time of their mastectomy or later (their address and telephone number are on page 195).

Different opinions about treatment

The form of treatment your consultant proposes will partly depend on the type of cancer, and where it is found. Most breast cancers are limited to a well-defined lump but some may have an area of thickening instead. A mammogram may show a 'suspicious area' elsewhere in the breast and in some cases the cancer may be attached to the chest muscle. These differences don't necessarily mean that the cancer is more serious but it does mean that more breast tissue (and possibly some underlying muscle) may need to be removed. Your surgeon can tell you if this is the case and between you, you can decide which surgical procedure will be most appropriate.

Which treatment is offered also depends on the preference of the surgeon. Doctors disagree about this question. Some favour breast conservation (partial mastectomy and lumpectomy) arguing that there is sufficient evidence that these treatments are effective in treating primary breast cancer if they are combined with radiotherapy. It also avoids the distress of losing a breast which can be very upsetting for some women.

Others remain unconvinced and say more long-term trials need to be assessed before a change in treatment is justified. They argue that the routine use of radiotherapy is undesirable because of its long-term effects. They also point out that partial mastectomy or lumpectomy are not without psychological problems themselves. Not all operations that conserve the breast have a good cosmetic result and some women will be preoccupied with worry about local recurrence in the breast.

Having the opportunity to choose

Given these differences of opinion within the medical profession, it is important that your consultant asks *your* opinion about which treatment or combination of treatments you feel happiest with. Each treatment has its advantages and disadvantages. Some women will prefer to have a mastectomy or lumpectomy with radiotherapy. Some women who choose mastectomy will want breast reconstruction and some women will prefer to leave well alone. The choices open to you will partly depend on the size of the cancer and whether there is other evidence of cancer in the breast. When you discuss the possible choices with your surgeon, keep reminding yourself that it is *your* body and *your* breast that is under discussion. One organization which has campaigned energetically for a change in approach to breast surgery in the Jeannie Campbell Radiotherapy Appeal. Particularly for early breast cancers, this organization gives advice and support for women who feel their choices are being limited to mastectomy. (See the Address list on page 195).

Some hospitals are involved in trial studies of different forms of surgery. This may mean that you are given less choice as a result so it is important to discuss with your consultant any trial arrangement in your hospital (see Chapter 7). It is also the case that some consultants will have more experience of one form of surgery which may influence their recommendations.

If you prefer your consultant to choose for you because you feel he has more experience, that's fine. If you feel strongly in favour of one treatment and your consultant favours another, discuss this with him and if he is unwilling to perform the operation you want, ask to be referred elsewhere. It is worth finding out which consultant in your area will be most sympathetic to your choice of treatment. Your GP or health visitor may be able to help you find this out or you can discuss this with the breast care nurse, if your local hospital has one. If you need to, enlist their support in ensuring that your wishes are acted upon.

The important thing is to give yourself time to adjust to your new situation so that you can come to a decision about which treatment you prefer. Chapters 13 and 14 will also help you to come to an informed choice.

Further reading

Michael Baum, *Breast Cancer — The Facts* (Oxford University Press, 1988) explains the different forms of mastectomy. In the book, Professor Baum is opposed to lumpectomy. He has since changed his opinion in the light of new evidence.

Sarah Boston and Jill Louw, *Disorderly breasts* (Camden Press, 1987) gives useful details on different forms of treatment.

Stephen Fulder, *How to Survive Medical Treatment: A holistic approach to the risks and side-effects of orthodox medicine* (Century Paperbacks, 1987).

Radiotherapy: your questions answered, Patient Information Series, Number Two, by the Patient Education Group, The Royal Marsden Hospital, 1986.

The Treatment of Primary Breast Cancer, Conference Papers, 1986, available from King's Fund College, 2 Palace Court, London W2 4HS. These papers cover all aspects of treatment for breast cancer. They tend to be written for a medical audience. They show the variation in opinion about different treatments including surgery and radiotherapy.

CHAPTER THIRTEEN
Surgery — what to expect

This chapter describes what is likely to happen when you go into hospital to have surgery for breast cancer.

The chapter starts by suggesting some ways you can prepare yourself for surgery and explains the tests you may be given beforehand. It looks at ways in which you can help to reduce the after-effects of different forms of surgery and things you can do to give yourself the best chance of a speedy recovery. It also briefly describes the different detachable breast forms which are available for women who have a mastectomy (or partial mastectomy).

The chapter ends by looking at the care and support that's available after the operation when you are in hospital and later on when you go home.

Preparing to go into hospital

There are several things you can do to make your stay in hospital less stressful. Some of these can be done before you go.

● Eat a healthy diet and get advice about vitamins along the lines suggested on page 93. Many people are deficient in vitamins and minerals and these are important in aiding the healing process. Vitamin C, Vitamin E, Vitamin B complex and zinc are particularly helpful in healing wounds. Even if you only change your diet or start to take a vitamin and mineral supplement a week beforehand, it will help

● Choose some personal things to take with you — photographs, a shawl, perfume — anything which makes you feel more at home while you're in hospital

● Hospital food is often unappetizing and stodgy so take in some healthy snacks. Organize friends and relatives to bring in tasty things to eat. A fresh fruit salad, a freshly squeezed orange and grapefruit drink, a home-made soup or a small plate of your favourite dish will lighten your spirits and help your recovery

● Take a personal stereo (try to borrow one if you haven't already got one) to listen to your favourite tapes when you're feeling low or can't sleep. Buy or make your own relaxation tape before you go into hospital. Doing a relaxation exercise can help to calm you when anxiety seems to get the upper hand (see page 155)

● Take something you enjoy doing, like reading a book or knitting, something that you will find restful to do and which takes your mind off your worries

● Take a note-pad and a pen. You might want to write down your thoughts and feelings about what is happening to you. It sometimes helps to ease a troubled mind and helps you to feel more in control. It's also helpful to jot down any questions you want to ask the doctor

● Take plenty of change for the telephone and for small treats from the hospital trolley or shop.

Getting support

Most women undergo treatment for breast cancer before they've fully taken in their diagnosis. Anxiety about their health and their future may be uppermost in their minds when they reach hospital. To have to then go through surgery and possibly radiotherapy or other treatments may be frightening. In this situation it is important to have as much personal support as possible.

We can find that support in many different ways. It may be a partner, an old friend or close relative, or sometimes one of the nursing staff. Whoever it is, if at all possible, find someone you can turn to when you need to during this time — someone who will support you in your decisions, listen to your needs and comfort you when you feel upset.

Breast care or breast counselling nurses An increasing number of hospitals have a breast care nurse who has special responsibility for women with breast cancer. She may visit you before you go into hospital and will come to see you again before the operation. Her job isn't to replace the nurses on the ward. She is there to try and answer any queries you have during treatment and to give you some support when you go home.

Local support groups In some areas there are local breast cancer support groups (sometimes mastectomy support groups) who visit women before and after they have had surgery to share experiences and offer support. Many women find it very useful to talk to another woman who has gone through surgery herself.

> Soon after the operation I was visited by a young woman from the support clinic who had a mastectomy seven years before and looked radiantly healthy and fit. She was very encouraging.

Other professional workers Another professional who may be able to help you is the medical social worker. You can ask to see her if you have any worries about work, financial problems, child-care and other family matters. But the nursing staff on the ward are often the ones who are there when you most need someone to talk to. Even if they seem busy, don't be afraid to let them know if you're feeling upset or depressed — they are there to care for your emotional as well as your physical needs.

The important thing is to use these different avenues of support when you need them. Between them, they can help you through this difficult time.

Preparing yourself for the operation

Everybody feels anxious before an operation, but you will feel more at ease and in control of your situation if you can be well-informed, well-nourished and well-rested. Here are some suggestions that may help.

Queries about the operation When you go into hospital for surgery the consultant or senior registrar and the anaesthetist will visit you to explain your operation and what to expect afterwards. Use these opportunities to discuss any worries you have. Ask to see the consultant a second time if you still have doubts about your choice of treatment. Here are some questions you may wish to ask:

● When am I going to theatre?

● What side-effects should I expect from the anaesthetic and the surgery?

● Are there any complications which I need to know about before I sign the consent form?

● How will I be cut and what will the wound look like afterwards?

- Will I have a drainage tube from the wound?
- Will I need a drip?
- How long will I be in theatre?
- How long will the wound take to heal?
- When will I be able to go home?

Studies have found that patients who are well informed about their operations are less anxious and afraid. This means that they have fewer side-effects from the anaesthetic and recover more quickly from the operation.

Queries about hospital routine You may have other queries about how the ward is organized, the rules about visiting and the choice of hospital food. The ward sister will be able to answer many of these questions:

- Can I stick up a picture or some photographs above my bed or on the side of my locker?
- Will I be moved during my stay in hospital?
- When can I have visitors during the day?
- Can my partner or close friend stay in the evening if I'm feeling anxious?
- Can I go outside if I'm feeling up to it?
- Is it possible to have my partner or close friend with me before I go to theatre and when I arrive back in the ward?
- Can I have fresh fruit with my meals?
- Is there wholemeal bread?
- Are there specific menus available for my religious or ethnic group? (Quite a few hospitals now have these menus but you may need to ask — staff may not think to tell you about them.)
- Is there a vegetarian menu?

The majority of nurses, from the ward sister to the nursing auxiliary, will want to make you feel as comfortable as possible while you are in hospital and will be sympathetic and helpful to any requests you make.

I was in a pleasant modern ward. My bed was by a window with a view of a small garden below. Nursing staff were very pleasant and helpful but the ward was obviously understaffed. Amenities were good — several bathrooms and loos, food ordered daily from menu sheets, always with vegetarian dishes available and fresh fruit. Library trolley, WVS 'shop' trolley, portable phone, radio headphones, etc.

Things to help you rest and relax Breathing and relaxation exercises can help to reduce anxiety and make you feel more relaxed. This can be particularly helpful before going to sleep and before going to theatre. It may mean that you don't need a sleeping pill or tranquillizing drug before the anaesthetic (see page 117).

Aromatic oils like rosemary (relaxes tense muscles) and peppermint (aids digestion and loosens tension) can be used to massage the skin, or you can just smell their fragrance. These essential oils can also be taken by mouth in very small quantities (one or two drops in a glass of water, four times a day). Women who use aromatic oils find them soothing and relaxing.

Herb teas can also help. If you're having a problem getting to sleep, cut out coffee and tea in the evening and try drinking camomile tea instead. (You can bring a packet of camomile tea bags with you and ask the nurse to make you up a cup rather than take a sleeping tablet which may leave you groggy in the morning.)

Traditional or complementary practitioners can suggest other herbal and homoeopathic remedies to help you relax and minimize the side-effects of treatment but it's wise to check to see if any self-medication conflicts with hospital treatment.

Tests and procedures

When you are admitted you may be given a blood test, a urine test and four-hourly temperature, pulse and blood pressure checks. The four-hourly chart is kept at the foot of your bed and you may like to check this every so often while you're in hospital. These are routine tests and provide information which will help the doctors to decide on any medication.

For reasons of space patients are asked to send their clothes home. (You will have a bedside locker for your personal things.) You might like to keep some clothes with you — a scarf or a cardigan to brighten up your appearance and your spirits.

Soon after you arrive in hospital a doctor will come and ask you for details about your medical history. This information will go into your hospital notes. (Patients aren't usually allowed to look at these notes but you can ask your GP, if she is willing, to send for them once you leave hospital and let you see them.)

You may be given a chest X-ray or a bone or liver scan to check for any stray cancer cells in the liver and the bones. This doesn't mean your consultant thinks the cancer has spread. In some hospitals these tests are part of the routine procedure for all patients with cancer.

A bone or liver scan is taken by injecting a small amount of radioactive liquid into a vein. More radioactivity goes to abnormal tissue and this is detected on scanning equipment. A liver scan can also be done by using ultrasound equipment (see Chapter 9).

The information contained in the X-ray or scan can be helpful either to reassure you that the cancer hasn't spread, or to give you and your consultant the necessary information to plan further treatment.

Signing the consent form

Before any operation, patients are asked to sign a form agreeing to surgery and a general anaesthetic. This form may include clauses which you want to query or delete. It's important to give yourself time to read the consent form carefully so that you can think about what you're agreeing to and discuss it with your visitors. As was pointed out earlier, women who have a frozen section biopsy should give clear instructions about any further treatment. It's worth remembering that your consultant is required to give you a clear explanation of any treatment proposed and should only proceed after you have been fully counsulted. So if you are unhappy about any wording in the form, query it with your consultant and, if necessary, cross out any words you're not happy with before signing it.

What to expect from surgery

Going to the theatre You will not be able to eat or drink anything on the day of your operation. A notice saying 'nil by mouth' or something similar will be put above your bed to avoid mistakes. This is to minimize the possibility of being sick from the anaesthetic. A nurse will probably shave your armpit on the side where the operation is to be performed.

Waiting to go to theatre is a time when a relaxation exercise, listening to your favourite tape, or some comforting words may help you to relax.

An hour or so before surgery you may be given a tranquillizer or pre-med. The pre-med might make your mouth and throat dry.

If you are able to relax, you may feel you don't need this. You may also be given a drug to stop you vomiting as a result of the general anaesthetic.

You will be taken to theatre on a trolley, usually by a nurse from your ward. The anaesthetist usually greets you and gives you the anaesthetic by injection (normally into a vein on the back of your hand) just before you go into theatre. The drugs relax the muscles as well as putting you to sleep. (The anaesthetist may ask you to start counting — most people are asleep before they reach ten!) During surgery the anaesthetist will give a further gas anaesthetic which will last for the rest of the operation. An airway tube is put down your throat, which might feel a little sore because of this. Your shoulder may also feel sore after the operation because while you are asleep the arm on the side of the breast to be operated on is tied to an arm rest at right angles to the body. This gives the surgeon a good view of the breast and the armpit. The size and shape of the wound will depend on the form of surgery you are having. (See figure 9).

The after-effects of the operation

Recovering after the operation is the first step in recovering good health. If you know what to expect it helps to prepare you for any unpleasant after-effects. Most of these pass very quickly and can be helped by medication. Herbal and homoeopathic remedies may also be helpful.

Dizziness and sickness Most people feel a bit dazed and woozy when they 'come to' after an operation. Some women are sick or feel nauseous. Some have a very dry throat. These symptoms usually last one or two days. Feelings of weariness and fatigue can last several days.

Pain and discomfort After surgery, the area around the stitches will be swollen and bruised and, in the case of mastectomy, one or two drainage tubes will add to the discomfort. These tubes are removed in about four or five days.

Some women are far more sensitive to pain than others. They may have pain down the side of the body, in the armpit or in the back. If you are in pain, don't hesitate to tell the nurse. In most cases, once the wound has settled down a little, the pain should go, apart from some soreness which may last a little longer.

Tissue removed   Cut/scar

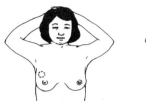 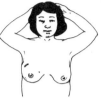

Lumpectomy. The surgeon makes a cut parallel to the circle around the nipple. This leaves a neater scar than a cut across the breast towards the nipple.

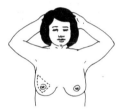 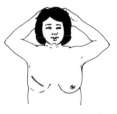

Partial mastectomy. This is a larger cut. If the lump is near the armpit, one cut will be sufficient to remove the lump and take a sample of lymph nodes. Otherwise two cuts will be made.

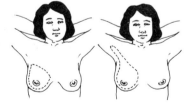 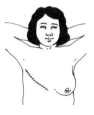

Different forms of mastectomy. This partly depends on where the lump is and whether some or all of the lymph nodes are removed. This is the most usual cut.

Figure 9 What the cut will look like.

The modern drugs used to control pain after the operation are very effective but some women experience drowsiness which can add to feelings of anxiety and depression. If this worries you, you may prefer to use herbal and homoeopathic remedies, and breathing and relaxation exercises to relieve pain.

> Some homoeopathic remedies do seem to help you get over an operation more quickly. I took arnica which is meant to help swelling, bruising and pain and I'm sure it helped me.

It's a good idea to see a traditional or complementary practitioner about remedies for pain relief before you go into hospital if you'd like to use them and it's wise to inform hospital staff of your choice.

Other side-effects Women who have had a mastectomy may also experience a tightness and numbness where the cut has been made. Others complain of more generalized numbness or pins and needles in the area of the breast, in their arms and in their fingers on the side of the operation. (Some of these sensations can take months to fade completely.) Some women also have an itching sensation which feels as if it won't go away. This is due to nerve endings settling down after surgery. Unexpected pain, months after the wound has healed, can also be caused by nerve endings growing again but this will settle down.

Practical suggestions to counter these side-effects

Many of the suggestions made earlier about preparing for an operation apply equally well after the event.

Some studies have shown that using mental imagery of the healing process can help you recover more quickly. Try to visualize a positive image of your body recovering and being healed. For example, you might imagine yourself lying in a garden on a lovely summer's day, the sun warming your body and healing your breast or you might imagine lots of little immune system workers busily doing overtime to mend the wound. While you're relaxing your mind and your body, imagine your own version of healing. This can give you a sense of well-being and many women have found it helpful.

Wheat-germ oil or evening primrose oil can help in healing of surgical wounds and can lessen scarring. It has also been found that wheat-germ oil can be used long after surgery to help to soften any scarring, particularly keloid scars, and this can help to improve the appearance of the scar.

Length of stay in hospital

Women having a lumpectomy normally stay in hospital for three days and return a week later to have the stitches removed. The length of stay in hospital will vary for women who have mastectomy. It will normally be about a week or ten days. The stitches may be removed while you're in hospital or later in an outpatient clinic.

Arm and shoulder exercises after surgery

Special exercises will help you get back full movement in your arm and shoulder after breast surgery. This helps to stop any

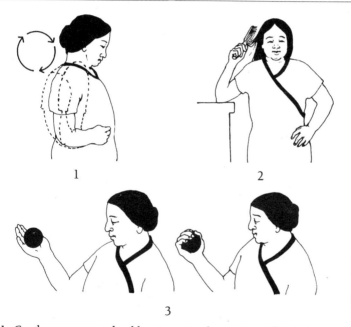

1. *Gently rotate your shoulders in a circular motion.* This helps to loosen the muscles in the area of your chest and your shoulders.

2. *Brush your hair using the arm on the side of the operation.* If you need to, rest your elbow on the locker beside your bed.

3. *Gently squeeze a soft object in your hand and then relax.* Repeat this a few times but stop if it begins to hurt.

Figure 10 Three simple shoulder exercises

stiffness in your shoulder. It is particularly important to regain full movement in the area if the lymph nodes or underlying chest muscle have been removed. These exercises help to establish a new 'balance' in the remaining muscles in the shoulder and arm if some chest muscle has been removed.

Usually a physiotherapist will come and explain each exercise to you while you are in hospital and may give you a sheet of exercises to take home.

> On the first day after the operation we were visited by a very jolly young physiotherapist who gave us arm exercises and impressed on us the importance of practising them regularly.

Figure 10 illustrates three exercises you can use while you're in hospital if no physiotherapist comes to see you. You should start gently and gradually build up the time you spend doing each exercise.

It's a good idea not to push yourself too hard to begin with so only do each exercise for as long as it is comfortable for you.

Later you can try more energetic chest and shoulder exercises. These are shown in Figure 11.

1. *Walking your hands up the wall.* Facing a wall, pat your hands gradually up the wall as far as you can and back again. Do this a few times each day for as long as is comfortable. Try marking your progress on the wall to give you encouragement.

2. *Clasping your arms behind your neck.* Standing with your legs slightly apart for balance, stretch your arms out sideways and then reach behind your neck and, if you can, clasp your hands.

3. *Swinging your arm.* Take some string and attach it to a door handle. Gently swing your arm, pulling on the string at the same time.

4. *Reaching behind your back.* Stretch your arms out sideways. Then bend your arms downwards and reach behind your back so that your hands meet.

5. *Bean bag exercises.* Use a pound of beans or lentils. With your right hand, drop the bag over your right shoulder and catch it in your left hand. Do this several times using both arms. Also throw the bean bag from hand to hand, with your arms bent.

6. *Pulling exercise.* Sit with your legs either side of an open door and put a skipping rope over the top of the door. Pull down gradually your good side, lifting the other arm up. Gently lower the arm and repeat.

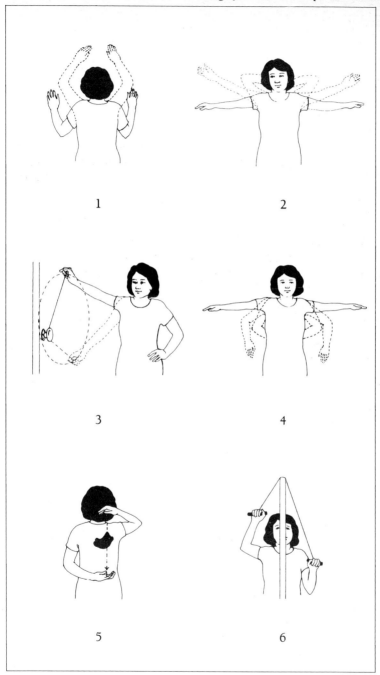

Figure 11 More shoulder and chest exercises

Begin by doing each exercise once and then gradually increase the number of times you do them. There's no set number. Each woman will be able to judge for herself what she is able to do. If you have any problems, contact the physiotherapist at the hospital.

Detachable breast forms

Before you go home, the breast care nurse or a specialist fitter will come to see you to discuss having a detachable breast form or prosthesis to take home with you. These fit into your bra and give you the appearance of having two breasts. Prostheses come in a range of sizes, weights and textures. They are washable and replaceable and several are obtainable on the NHS. While the wound is healing, you will be offered a lightweight stuffing for your bra. Later you will be given an appointment to fit a more substantial prosthesis. Many women worry that they'll have to buy special bras and clothes. This isn't the case. A prosthesis can fit into most makes of bra and no one will know the difference.

> I've been wearing a prosthesis for 10 years. I wouldn't feel dressed without it. There are loads of different types and it's taken me some time to find the one I wear now. I go swimming and wear bikinis like everyone else. It's okay.

Some women have mixed feelings about wearing a prosthesis. They don't feel it belongs so can't get used to it.

> They gave me a thing but I never really got into wearing it. I used to keep it in the linen cupboard. One day a friend who was staying said: 'Do you know there's a piece of chicken breast in amongst your towels?' I had a really good laugh and suddenly found I'd got enough sense of humour about my illness to throw it away and stop worrying about being lopsided.

A prosthesis solves the immediate problem of how we appear to the world but coming to terms with the personal grief of losing a breast and learning to live with a physically different body is part of a far longer process. We shall consider this in Chapter 19.

Looking after yourself when you go home

Before you leave hospital, you will be given an appointment for a post-operative check-up. This may include removing stitches if this hasn't already been done. You may also have a list of exercises to do at home.

Women who have had their lymph nodes removed (or irradiated) will be given advice on how to care for the arm on the side of the surgery. Because the lymphatic system may be weakened in that arm, you should avoid carrying heavy bags. It's also important to avoid having blood pressure taken or having an injection in the affected arm. This increases the possibility of swelling and fluid imbalance.

You can protect your hand and arm from cuts, scratches and pin pricks by wearing gardening gloves in the garden, rubber gloves if you're using a metal pot scourer or (wire wool) and by using a thimble when you're sewing. These reduce the possibility of infection which can be more problematic if all the lymph nodes in the armpit have been removed.

Other precautions include an electric razor if you shave beneath your arms and resting your arm on a pillow if it becomes swollen. If you do get a cut or scratch, it's wise to clean it well with antiseptic.

Not all women get lymphoedema but it's a possibility if you have had all your lymph nodes removed or have had radiotherapy in the area of the armpit (see comments on page 132).

Going home can be a difficult time of adjustment. Many women feel pleased to leave hospital, but they may also feel a bit apprehensive about going home. It means adjusting to a new situation and picking up the threads of your life. It can mean being thrown back on your own resources just when you are feeling rather vulnerable and lonely, after the bustle of the ward and the support of the nurses.

> I went home to the new house but it was obviously more than I could cope with so I went to stay with my sister. I still had some pain and slept badly. I'm sure I was suffering from shock after going into hospital for what I expected to be minor surgery. There was also a feeling of insecurity at being thrown back into the real world after being in the hospital, surrounded day and night by medical staff.
>
> My sister's GP and his nurse were amazingly supportive and saw me every day to check on the wounds — the armpit was slightly septic — and two weeks later I felt a good deal more human and though still feeling weak, I went home to start putting life in order again.

It's not unusual to feel upset or depressed after you go home, and it's a good idea to think about who you can turn to for support during these first weeks. Family and friends will be important but some women will want to go elsewhere to talk about their feelings and fears. If your hospital has a breast care nurse, she will visit you at home and give you some support in working through your feelings about having cancer. Community nurses, health visitors and your GP can also help.

Some women turn to a cancer support group (in some areas there are mastectomy support groups) where you can share your fears and feelings about having breast cancer with other women in the same situation. You may be given an address of a local group by the hospital. But there are also national organizations which can help with any enquiries about cancer and about support for women with cancer. Some useful addresses can be found on page 195.

It's important to persevere in looking for support and any information you need to help you renew your life. It may mean going to a counsellor or therapist, joining a group or relying on a good friend. It may also mean taking up new interests and commitments. Chapter 19 will discuss in greater detail the problems involved in adjusting to living with breast cancer and healing the psychological as well as the physical scars. A full list of cancer support organizations can be found on page 195.

Further reading

Michael Baum, *Breast Cancer: The Facts* (Oxford University Press, 1988) explains different forms of surgery.

Stephen Fulder, *How to Survive Medical Treatment: a holistic approach to the risks and side-effects of orthodox medicine* (Century Paperbacks, 1987) gives many useful suggestions, some of which have been described in this chapter.

Betty Westgate, *Coping with Breast Cancer* (The Breast Care and Mastectomy Association, 1987).

See also Chapter 19 for other suggestions.

CHAPTER FOURTEEN

Radiotherapy — what to expect

In Britain radiotherapy is rarely used on its own to treat primary breast cancer. It is mainly used to back up surgery where it is thought necessary. You may or may not be offered it, depending on the type of surgery and the location of the cancer (see Chapter 12).

This chapter explains how and when radiotherapy is likely to be given. It makes some suggestions on how to prepare yourself for treatment and describes what to expect when having it. The chapter ends by making some suggestions on how best to counter the after-effects of radiotherapy.

The procedure of radiotherapy

Radiotherapy usually begins about a month after surgery when the wound has healed. Not all hospitals have radiation equipment. If you live in a large city, there will be at least one hospital in your area which specializes in radiotherapy, but if you live out of town, you might have to travel some distance for treatment. This may involve staying in an NHS hostel while you have it. Your consultant will arrange this.

Treatment is usually several times a week, excluding weekends. Each session lasts roughly half an hour but only a few minutes of this involves exposure to radiation. The length of treatment will vary but it usually lasts four to six weeks. This will depend on the amount of radiation your doctors think you need and how much you should have each day. In the case of lumpectomy this basic treatment may be followed later by a 'booster' dose to the area where the lump was.

There are two ways of giving radiotherapy for breast cancer. The most usual way involves beaming high energy rays into the breast tissue or surrounding area. It may be necessary to do this from a number of different angles — these are carefully worked out beforehand. On your first visit, detailed X-rays may be taken and radiotherapy may not begin until after the second visit. A second method uses radioactive needles (see 'Booster treatment' below). With both methods, any radioactivity in the body disappears once the treatment is finished.

Radiotherapy can be used with all forms of surgery but opinions about its use have changed over the years. It is now felt that with mastectomies, particularly with radical and modified radical mastectomies, radiotherapy is not always necessary. But in some areas old practices die hard. If you have had a radical mastectomy and you are then offered radiotherapy, you may like to get a second opinion as another consultant may not think it necessary. With surgery which conserves the breast (lumpectomy and partial mastectomy) radiotherapy is used to lessen the chances of local recurrence.

Preparing for radiotherapy

Finding out about the treatment

Given that radiotherapy has both advantages and disadvantages for women (see Chapter 12), it's worth thinking through the pros and cons and discussing them with your surgeon and radiologist so that you can make an informed choice about radiotherapy, and feel confident in your decision to have it.

Here are some questions you might like to ask the radiologist before you agree to have treatment:

- What part of the breast tissue is going to be irradiated?
- If the lymph nodes are irradiated, am I likely to get fluid retention in my arm or my breast?
- What dose of radiotherapy will I be given?
- How many visits will I make over how many months?
- Is my skin likely to burn?
- What can I do to protect myself from skin burns?
- How will radiation affect my immune system?
- How long will any soreness or dry skin last after treatment finishes?
- How long will the tiredness last?

- Will my skin become discoloured?
- Will my breast feel different after radiotherapy?
- Will there be any long-term effects?

Most radiologists will be happy to discuss any aspect of treatment with you and it's important that you settle any doubts before you begin your treatment.

Things you can do for yourself

There are several things you can do to prepare yourself for radiotherapy, some of which will help to minimize its side-effects.

Keep up a healthy diet, and seek advice on vitamin supplements. Radiotherapy destroys several vitamins in the body, so it is particularly important to repair any vitamin deficiency. Increased consumption of vitamins and minerals can also help your body protect itself from the side-effects of radiotherapy. For example vitamin A, vitamin C and vitamin E are all affected by radiotherapy and these vitamins are important in healing body tissue. Trials using vitamin A and vitamin C have shown a decrease in numbers suffering side-effects of radiotherapy. You could ask your GP or consultant radiologist to prescribe vitamin supplements or seek help from a trained nutritionist (see page 194).

Prepare yourself mentally for radiotherapy. It is now recognized that patients who use mental imagery when they have radiotherapy or chemotherapy tend to have fewer side-effects and tend to benefit more from their treatment. It can take time to think of a suitable image so try working one out beforehand. For example, some women visualize the radiation rays as soldiers fighting any remaining cancer cells and other women imagine their radiotherapy as floodwaters cleansing and clearing away cancer cells. Choose an image which suits you so that while you have your radiotherapy you can concentrate on it and make it work for you.

Some women have found that using a mental image which shields them from the effects of radiotherapy has stopped soreness or burning of the skin. For example, imagine that you are lying on a beach with some good quality sun tan lotion on while the radiation beam is on. Other women have found hypnosis useful before having radiotherapy. However outlandish it appears, convincing the body that you won't have side-effects does seem to work for many people. (See *Getting Well Again* in the reading list for more ideas about mental images.)

Explain the likely side-effects of radiotherapy to your family and friends (see Chapter 12). You may feel tired and lacking in energy as a result of treatment. They should know this so that they can help you to rest and relax (by looking after children, cooking or doing some shopping for you, for example). It's also important that they realize that you may feel depressed from your treatment. Knowing that this is a side-effect of radiotherapy can make it easier for you to face it.

Think out ways of coping with depression. This may mean giving yourself special treats, being comforted when you feel upset and it may mean seeking professional help from a counsellor or psychotherapist if you feel really down

Look out or borrow some clothes which won't irritate the area of the breast while you're having radiotherapy and while your skin is sore. Silk is sometimes suggested and you might be able to find a small piece of silk to make a simple silk bodice to wear, to stop any rubbing. If this isn't possible, choose loose clothes with soft material which won't chafe too much as you move — like a baggy T-shirt, for example

Make contact with women in your area who have had radiotherapy. You may be able to do this through contacting a local cancer self-help group. The Breast Care and Mastectomy Association can also put you in touch with women who are willing to share their experiences of radiotherapy (see address on page 195)

Try something new while you do radiotherapy. Treatment only takes a small amount of time each day and you may find that you have time on your hands. Perhaps start an adult education class or sort out the family photograph album — something that isn't too taxing and is enjoyable enough to take your mind off things

Finally, you might like to ask to see the room where you will have radiotherapy when you go for your first appointment. You may be able to meet the radiographer who will operate the machinery and ask what the procedure will be. Radiotherapy machinery is large and a bit intimidating. It may help you to relax on the day if you know what the equipment is like and how it works.

What to expect at treatment sessions

Before radiotherapy begins your breast will be marked with ink to show where the radiation beam should go. These marks remain while you're having treatment so it's important not to wipe them off by mistake. You may be told not to wash the area which will be irradiated because this increases the possibility of soreness or the breakdown of the skin. Or you may be told that you can gently sponge the area and dab it dry, being careful to avoid rubbing it with a coarse towel. It means you cannot have a shower and must be very careful when you wash or have a bath. It also means you can't use deodorants or perfumes in the area. You should only use baby powder.

Treatment takes place in a hospital room where the radiographer will show you the equipment to be used. This consists of a special bed or couch, attached to which will be a large machine from which the beam of radiation will come. The machine will rotate around you if radiotherapy is required at different angles. You will be asked to undress to the waist and lie down on the bed.

The radiographer will explain in what position she wants you to lie and she will take great care to make sure this is exactly right. She may use a measuring instrument made of perspex to help position where the beam will go. Once this is done, the radiographer goes into an adjoining room so that she is protected from radiation while radiotherapy is taking place. You will probably be able to talk to each other and she will be able to see you through a window in the wall. You have to stay very still for about two minutes while the beam of radiation is on. It will take slightly longer if the beam is used at different angles.

Before or during treatment, you might be given an X-ray using a special machine called a simulator. This checks the path of the radiotherapy and makes sure there is no unnecessary damage to surrounding tissue, such as the lungs.

Booster treatment

Women who have a lumpectomy or partial mastectomy may be given a booster dose of radiotherapy to the site of the operation. This is usually done using radiotherapy machinery but in some hospitals radioactive needles are used. (You will be given an anaesthetic while this is done.) These are threaded through the breast tissue where the cancer was lodged and are left in position for three or four days. Your breast may feel sensitive and a bit painful in the area of the implanted material. While the needles are in position, you will spend most of the time alone. Nursing staff and visitors have to limit the time they spend with you because of the radioactive material in your breast. Children and pregnant women are not allowed to see you. So it's a good idea to think up things to take in with you to help pass the time if you decide to have this form of booster treatment.

Reducing any side-effects

Radiotherapy does have side-effects, but don't let these become a self-fulfilling prophecy. Most women *don't* experience difficulties and most side-effects can be minimized by careful preparation, sensible precautions while having treatment and continuing to look after yourself when the treatment has finished.

If your skin does become sore and break down, the hospital may use gentian violet to dry the skin or prescribe a cortisone cream. Traditional and complementary practitioners tend to argue that prevention is better than cure. They may suggest you use a cream or lotion before, during and after treatment. Wheat-germ oil is helpful in healing burns or wounds and Aloe vera gel is good for radiation burns.

Fibrosis in the breast area and in the lung is more difficult to correct. Firmer breast tissue sometimes settles down after a few months but fibrous bands of tissue may remain permanently and any fibrosis in the lungs will be permanent. Traditional and complementary therapists may be able to help improve this.

If the lymph nodes in the armpit are irradiated, care is taken to leave some lymph nodes to prevent lymphoedema or fluid retention. This isn't always possible. There will be a weakness in that arm and care should be taken to protect the arm and minimize swelling along the lines suggested on page 124. There may be some fluid retention in the breast but this normally goes within about a year or so as the tissue settles down.

If you experience any long-term pain as a result of radiotherapy, acupuncture may be able to help. Other possibilities are herbal and homoeopathic remedies and hypnosis, all of which have had some success with pain relief.

Having radiotherapy means you will need to take good care of yourself and your health. A healthy diet and vitamin supplements, relaxation and rest and mental imagery can all help the possible side-effects of treatment. The ideas suggested in this chapter should help you to feel confident and in control of your treatment and its effects on you.

Further reading

Sarah Boston and Jill Louw, *Disorderly Breasts* (Camden Press, 1987).

Stephen Fulder, *How to Survive Medical Treatment: a holistic approach to the risks and side-effects of orthodox medicine* (Century Paperbacks, 1987). This gives useful suggestions on the use of traditional and complementary treatments to minimize side effects, some of which are used in the chapter.

O. Carl Simonton, M.D., Stephanie Matthews Simouton and James L. Creighton, *Getting Well Again,* (Bantam Books, 1980).

Radiotherapy: your questions answered, Patient Information Series, Number Two, The Patient Education Group, The Royal Marsden Hospital, 1987.

CHAPTER FIFTEEN

Assessing the seriousness of breast cancer — making a prognosis

Modern medicine is now able to assess different kinds of cancer and the possibility of cancer spread. This chapter explains the methods which are used by doctors to assess the seriousness of the disease so that they can plan any follow-up treatment. However, cancer is an unpredictable disease and doctors can only give an informed guess about the future.

The shock of discovering breast cancer makes many women fear the worst. They think that they will die within months of treatment and some women expect to die during surgery. *This is very unlikely indeed.* You have already learnt that there are different types of breast cancer. Some cancers can be completely cured and others can be successfully controlled for many years.

Not all women will want to seek an opinion about the type of cancer they have, whether it is fast or slow growing or the possibility of cancer spread. They will prefer to leave that in the lap of the gods and get on with their lives. If you would rather do this and rely on the experience and expertise of your consultant, that's fine. It is for this reason that this separate chapter has been put aside, to give you the choice of reading it. So you may like to pause here, before deciding to read on.

Different ways of assessing the seriousness of breast cancer

Doctors, using the skills of biochemists, cytologists and radiologists look for several pointers in making their assessment:

● They measure the size of the cancerous growth. The smaller the size, the more likely it is to be an early cancer. Small cancers can also mean slow-growing cancers but this doesn't depend on size alone

● They study a sample of the lymph nodes from the armpit and sometimes from the centre of the chest. This allows them to 'stage' the cancer depending on how many lymph nodes contain stray cancer cells. Early cancers or cancers that are unlikely to spread to other parts of the body are less likely to have cancer cells in any of the lymph nodes

● They study the structure and behaviour of the cancer cells to see how much they have altered from normal cells. This study is called histologic assessment. Cancers are graded depending on whether they are 'well differentiated', 'moderately differentiated' or 'poorly differentiated' (see Chapter 4 for more information about cell behaviour and cell differentiation)

● Finally doctors look to see if the cancer cells are sensitive to hormones, particularly to oestrogen. This may also give an indication of how much the cells have changed. Many normal breast cells are sensitive to a number of hormones as we have seen. Some cancer cells appear to lose this capacity. Scientists aren't sure how important this is but it seems clear that cancers that haven't lost any of their sensitivity may be more responsive to hormone related drugs (see Chapter 16 and 19).

The size and the stage of the cancer is partly dependent on time. This is why women are encouraged to report any change in their breasts as early as possible. Early treatment increases the possibility of cure. Information about cell differentiation and hormone sensitivity tells doctors whether the cancer is likely to spread and whether it is possible to reduce the growth rate. It is on the basis of this knowledge that follow-up treatment is recommended (see Chapter 16).

Questions you might like to ask your consultant

Assessing the seriousness of breast cancer gives us information which may affect not only our choice of treatment but also our priorities in the way we organize our lives. Knowing how this assessment is made enables us to ask for information which we might otherwise not be told. With this information we can plan our own whole-person treatment programme which may include traditional and complementary choices as well as the treatments modern medicine has to offer.

Here are some questions you might like to ask:

● How large is the cancer? (Has your consultant any comment to make about this?)

● Is there any lymph node involvement? How many lymph nodes are affected? (Has your consultant any comment to make about this?)

● What sort of cells havé been found? How well differentiated. are they?

● Are the cells sensitive to hormones or not?

● What treatments will be most effective in treating my particular cancer?

Accurate knowledge about what sort of cancer you have can give you greater confidence in any treatments you decide upon. Knowledge can help to give you some control over what is happening. It can help you find the confidence to voice your opinions and get actively involved in decisions about your follow-up treatment. Most women will be guided by the choices their hospital consultant suggests. A few women will choose traditional and complementary medicine instead and an increasing number of women will want to combine modern and alternative therapies.

Further reading

There is little popular literature which discusses the staging of breast cancer. Papers prepared for the King's Fund Conference on *The Treatment of Primary Breast Cancer* held in 1986 are helpful but are quite technical. These can be obtained from King's Fund College, 2 Palace Court, London W2 4HS.

CHAPTER SIXTEEN
Follow-up treatments for breast cancer

Once your consultant has made an assessment of the type of cancer you have and the stage it has reached, he may discuss the possibility of follow-up treatment. This will be considered if there is evidence of stray cancer cells in the lymph nodes or other signs that the cancer is likely to spread to another part of the body. This can be a frightening prospect but remember that some cancers grow extremely slowly and it may take decades before a secondary cancer (metastasis) develops, even if there is some evidence of cancer cells in the lymph nodes.

Long before any secondary cancer is found, tiny groups of cells can form (called micro-metastases) and it is these which follow-up treatments hope to eliminate. They also aim to control or slow down any further spread of cancer. Because these follow-up treatments affect cells throughout the body they are sometimes described as systemic treatments for breast cancer.

This chapter looks at the different choices of systemic treatment which modern medicine offers women when there is evidence of lymph node involvement. There are two approaches. The first approach attempts to limit the influence of hormones on cancer cells by disrupting the normal hormonal balance in the body. This is because hormones, in particular oestrogen, appear to influence the growth of breast cancers. The second approach uses cytotoxic drugs to poison cancer cells in the body, (cyto means cell, toxic means poisonous). The popular name for this is chemotherapy. This chapter describes these treatments and explains how each one works. It also looks at the advantages and disadvantages of each approach and suggests ways of minimizing side-effects which, in the case of chemotherapy, can sometimes be severe.

Your age and the type of cancer you have will influence which treatment you are offered. Medical science is divided about which approach is better so treatment varies from hospital to hospital. It can also depend on the preference of your consultant and whether a trial is being carried out (see Chapter 7). The chapter ends by discussing the choices of treatment open to women who have evidence of cancer in their lymph nodes.

Treatments which alter hormone activity in the body

Since the 1890s, scientists have recognized a connection between hormones circulating in the body and the development of breast cancer. What the connection is remains unclear but altering hormone levels in the body, particularly oestrogen levels, appears to help in controlling the growth of cancer.

During our reproductive years most breast cells continually receive hormone messages which alter their behaviour in the monthly cycle. The cells recognize these messages using a 'receptor' which looks out for hormone signals. Oestrogen receptors are continually watchful for signals so that when oestrogen levels rise, changes take place in breast tissue. After the menopause, oestrogen is still produced in the body and oestrogen receptors still look out for signals.

Most breast cancers have this ability to respond to oestrogen signals but some don't. Breast cancers can be assessed, therefore, according to whether they are sensitive to oestrogen. Doctors study cancer cells to see if they have oestrogen receptors or not (ER positive and ER negative for short — in the United States oestrogen is spelled estrogen and the 'e' best represents the initial sound).

Hormone-related treatments aim to restrict the influence of oestrogens so that oestrogen-sensitive cancer cells will be less active. These treatments appear to be most successful with cancers which are clearly ER positive, but sometimes even ER negative cancers respond to hormonal drugs.

Hormone-related treatments

There are three methods of limiting the influence of oestrogens. The first (which is only appropriate for women still having periods) uses surgery or radiotherapy to remove the ovaries. The second uses 'anti-oestrogen' drugs which prevent hormone-sensitive cells from reacting to oestrogen and the third method uses other drugs which alter the hormonal balance in some way. (These are discussed in Chapter 19.)

Surgery or radiotherapy of the ovaries The ovaries are the major producers of oestrogen during our fertile years so for women still having periods, removing the ovaries is a way of drastically reducing oestrogen levels. This can be done by surgery or radiotherapy.

Removing the ovaries (called oophorectomy) or irradiating the ovaries prolongs the time free of any recurrence of disease (called the disease-free interval) although survival in the long-term only seems to be improved in a few trial studies. Cutting off a supply of oestrogens from the ovaries is helpful but eventually the body is able to adapt itself and rely on increased oestrogen production elsewhere in the body. If this happens, hormone-related drugs may need to be used to limit the influence of oestrogen (see below and comments on drugs affecting the adrenal glands on page 183).

Anti-oestrogen drugs In recent years drugs have been developed which appear to attach themselves to the oestrogen receptors in the cells. When the receptor is 'occupied', the cell is unable to recognize or respond to oestrogen signals and so its behaviour remains unchanged. Scientists still don't know exactly how this happens because it seems that women with ER negative cancers can still benefit from these drugs, and some women with positive cancers don't seem to benefit at all.

The drug most widely used is tamoxifen (trade names are Nolvadex and Tamofen). This is taken in tablet form, usually on a daily basis. In different trial studies it has been given for one, two and up to five years and doctors are now considering the possibility of prescribing tamoxifen over longer periods. It takes about six months before any benefit is felt from the drug. In more advanced cases, some symptoms at first may get worse before they start to improve (see Chapter 19).

Anti-oestrogen drugs are relatively new so trials have not been going on long enough to test the drug's overall effectiveness but the results so far have been encouraging. Originally tamoxifen was only given to postmenopausal women with advanced cancers and in these cases it was found to reduce some secondary cancer growths (see Chapter 19). More recently it has been given as a follow-up treatment for early cancer to both premenopausal and postmenopausal women. Short-term trial results suggest that the drug increases the length of time before any recurrence of the disease and there has been a 30 per cent increase in the number of women surviving five years on. More trials over a longer period are needed before long-term benefits can be assessed.

Side-effects of hormone-related treatments and ways of reducing them

Hormones have a vital influence on the tissue of the breasts and in many other parts of the body (see Chapter 2). This is because hormones 'tell' cells how to behave. It is not surprising, then, that if hormone production is altered, changes will take place in the body.

Surgery or radiotherapy If the ovaries are removed or irradiated, the sudden drop in oestrogen and progesterone 'tells' the body that child-bearing is finished and a process similar to the menopause is set in motion within a few days of the operation.

Women's experience of the menopause varies greatly, and this is also true for women who have their ovaries removed or irradiated. Symptoms can include hot flushes, sweating, headaches, weight gain, vaginal dryness, water retention (a 'bloated' feeling), occasional growth of body hair and a tendency to calcium deficiency (this can result in brittle bones or osteoporosis). You may experience some of these if your ovaries are removed or irradiated. Most problems will settle down as the body adjusts to a new hormonal balance.

Anti-oestrogen drugs Anti-oestrogen drugs can also produce symptoms suggesting that the hormonal balance has been disrupted in the ovaries and elsewhere. Periods may stop. Some women may put on weight. Others have hot flushes and sweating. Less common symptoms are increased blood pressure, nausea, vaginal bleeding, lowering of the voice and calcium deficiency.

Any side-effects can be reduced by changing the dose and can be reversed by stopping the treatment.

All of the side-effects described above will benefit from developing a health programme which includes:

● A varied diet (including natural diuretics — see page 93)

● Vitamin supplements (Rosetta Reitz suggests 800 units of vitamin E complex and 2,000-3,000 milligrams of vitamin C for hot flushes and sweating — see Further reading, page 146)

● Breathing exercises, regular exercise and relaxation

● Some women also find herbal and homoeopathic remedies helpful and others have used acupuncture for menopausal symptoms.

Hormonal changes may leave some women feeling vulnerable and depressed. Symptoms can be unpredictable and younger women who have their ovaries removed or irradiated, have to come to terms with losing their fertility. Having some measure of control over your symptoms will help counter depression but grieving for the loss of your fertility may need the help and support of others. Your GP can recommend a counsellor or therapist and the national organizations listed on page 192 can put you in touch with support groups and individual women in your area who have faced similar problems.

Cytotoxic drugs: how they work and how they're given

Cytotoxic drugs are poisonous. Slower-growing cells are able to repair any damage but rapidly dividing cells fail to recover. Unlike radiotherapy, where the highest dose is aimed at the breast, high doses of cytotoxic drugs can reach all cells throughout the body. This explains the wide range of side-effects experienced with chemotherapy.

Scientists don't yet fully understand how cytotoxic drugs work. Some drugs seem to interfere with a cell's ability to grow (resulting in the death of cells) while other drugs seem to kill the cells outright. Because these drugs have different effects, a 'cocktail' of drugs is usually given.

Sometimes cytotoxic agents are combined with steroid drugs. It is thought that short-term use of steroids can help protect the bone marrow and influence the dividing phase of cells so that the chemotherapy is more effective. Steroid drugs can have serious side-effects if they are taken over a long period of time (see Chapter 19) but these will be minimal in the short term.

A programme of chemotherapy will be planned for six months or a year. During this time, one or more drugs will be given to you in hospital at regular intervals. Treatment takes several months because time is allowed for the body to recover a little between each treatment.

Cytotoxic drugs can be given in a number of different ways:

● In tablet form — you may also be given tablets to take home with you

● By injection into a muscle or under the skin. This will be done in outpatients and you will be able to go home afterwards

● Drugs can be fed into a vein either by injection or by using a drip. If a drip is used, you will have to stay in hospital for one or two nights.

During your treatment hospital staff will take great care to monitor the effects of the drugs and alterations will be made if the side-effects are severe.

Chemotherapy is usually given after surgery and radiotherapy has finished. In the past it was given when there was evidence of cancer spread. In the last few years, it has been given earlier in the hope of destroying any micro-metastases before they develop further. Some doctors even suggest that chemotherapy should be given immediately before surgery since they think that surgery may have the effect of encouraging micro-metastases to become active. While this has yet to be proved, chemotherapy given soon after surgery seems to be more effective.

The side-effects of chemotherapy and how to minimize them

Chemotherapy has a reputation for unpleasant side-effects but this won't necessarily be the case. Some women are affected more than others. Side-effects also depend on the drugs used and the dose given. If you do decide to have chemotherapy, try to keep an open mind and don't talk yourself into expecting to feel ill. It's important to start your treatment positively, reminding yourself that you have chosen this because it is going to help you. Ask your consultant what side-effects you can expect and prepare yourself for these. In a number of studies it has been found that a positive attitude lessens any side-effects of treatment.

A healthy diet and vitamin supplements will ensure that you're as well as possible before treatment begins (see suggestions on page 93). Mental imagery and hypnosis can also help before you start treatment and while you are having it.

Because cytotoxic drugs damage all fast growing cells, it is these cells which will produce symptoms of ill-health. These *may* include the following:

Mouth ulcers and infections. These can be eased by regular mouth-washes, careful brushing of teeth to avoid infections and small, light meals which are easily eaten. Avoid spicy meals and extremes of temperature. A natural antiseptic mouth-wash is glycerine and thymol

Feeling sick and vomiting. This is most likely immediately after treatment although some women also feel sick with anticipation before treatment begins. Hypnosis can be particularly helpful and eating small, light meals

Constipation and diarrhoea. Try to maintain a light diet and drink plenty of fluids. Also try to relax as much as possible

Hair loss (alopecia). Some but not all combinations of drugs can cause hair to fall out. If this is likely to happen, it's a good idea to cut your hair short before you start treatment. With some drugs, applying an ice pack round the head can help to reduce the likelihood of hair loss. Some women have found that using mental imagery has stopped their hair falling out

Hair loss can be inconvenient and unpredictable. Some women find wearing a hairnet useful, particularly at night. For women who lose their hair, wigs are available on the NHS and your own hair will grow back once treatment has finished. Many women report that their new head of hair is healthier than before treatment

Lowering the blood count. During chemotherapy you will be given regular blood tests to check the levels of red and white blood cells and platelets. (Platelets are smaller than ordinary blood cells and are important in healing.)

Blood cells are produced in the bone marrow. Chemotherapy depresses the levels of blood cells in the bone marrow and this can affect bleeding and bruising (which may be more noticeable while you're having treatment). It can also make you feel tired and run down. If the blood count falls below a safe level, treatment will be altered or a longer rest given between treatments so that you can recover. (The immune system soon recovers once chemotherapy has finished.)

Loss of periods and menopausal symptoms. Many women find that their periods stop during chemotherapy and some women experience menopausal symptoms of hot flushes, sweating, etc. In women over the age of 40 these changes are likely to be permanent. In younger women, periods will return once the treatment has finished

Weight gain. Some cytotoxic combinations encourage weight gain. Try to alter your diet if you notice yourself getting fatter. It may mean that you can have a different combination of drugs

Depression. Many women who have chemotherapy suffer from depression. Some side-effects can make you feel sick and unwell and losing your hair can be demoralizing. The combination of side-effects and the lowering of the blood count can make some women feel very depressed. Preparing yourself for chemotherapy and making sure you are well-rested, well-nourished and relaxed can help to lift feelings of depression. Writing about it can also help and, if necessary, you can seek help from a counsellor or psychologist. Most women find the depression begins to lift once treatment has finished. If steroids have been part of the treatment, this may take longer.

It is important to recognize that depression is a natural reaction to knowing you have cancer and to all the problems and uncertainties it brings. Coping with depression and learning to live with cancer is discussed further in Chapter 19.

Concern about chemotherapy and its side-effects

Since the early 1950s cytotoxic drugs have been used to treat cancer with some impressive results, for example, in the treatment of childhood leukaemia. Unpleasant side-effects have been seen as a necessary evil when the result is cure of the disease. With some other cancers, including breast cancer, the value of chemotherapy is less clear. In postmenopausal women, there is little evidence of long-term benefit although chemotherapy may improve cases of advanced breast cancer in the short term. Some doctors argue that any 'improvement' brought about by chemotherapy has to be balanced against the severity of the side-effects which some women experience. If the overall life-span is not significantly increased, some doctors argue that the quality of life is better without cytotoxic drugs and their side-effects.

For premenopausal women the picture is somewhat different. There is some evidence that about a quarter of the women in this group who have chemotherapy soon after any surgery will increase their survival time as a result of the treatment. The evidence suggests that those women who miss their periods during chemotherapy are the ones most likely to benefit.

Two explanations have been given for this difference between pre- and postmenopausal women. Doctors who advise chemotherapy believe that premenopausal women are able to tolerate higher (and therefore more effective) doses of toxic drugs than older women. Other doctors think it more likely that chemotherapy affects the ovaries and therefore limits the production of oestrogen in premenopausal women.

Research continues to try and improve the action of cytotoxic drugs while lessening their side-effects. One of the newest developments in chemotherapy involves the use of antibodies to 'deliver' the toxic chemical agents to the site of cancer cells (in the breast or elsewhere). Because the antibodies bind themselves to cancer cells rather than all fast growing cells, it is possible to concentrate the cytotoxic drugs around the cancer. This means lower doses can be given and used more effectively and it also means that side-effects should be reduced. This new treatment is in its early stages of development and so is not yet widely used.

The choices open to you

The type of treatment you are offered will depend on your age and on whether your cancer is hormone sensitive.

If you have passed the menopause, you are more likely to be offered tamoxifen than chemotherapy, because chemotherapy appears to be less effective in postmenopausal women. The exceptions to this will be where a trial is being run to test chemotherapy on older women, or where the cancer is ER negative and clearly unresponsive to tamoxifen. If you have passed the menopause and your consultant suggests chemotherapy to you, ask him what his reasons are for recommending it. It may be that you would prefer tamoxifen.

Premenopausal women may be offered the choice of chemotherapy, tamoxifen and other hormone-related treatments (oophorectomy or irradiation of the ovaries). In some hospitals, trials will be taking place to compare different treatments. If you have a preference, discuss this with your consultant. It may mean that you attend a different hospital for follow-up treatment.

Not all women will readily agree to follow-up treatments. A few will prefer to rely on traditional and complementary remedies instead. Others will want to combine modern treatments with traditional and complementary treatments. More and more women are using the self-help methods of visualization, relaxation, diet and meditation in treating breast cancer (see Chapter 17). All these decisions about treatment are complex and you may feel unable to assess the pros and cons and argue one way or the other. There can come a point when you simply wish to trust your chosen healers to do the best for you. Whatever your decision, it's important that you feel positive and have confidence in it.

Further reading

Michael Baum, *Breast Cancer: The Facts* (Oxford University Press, 1988).

Sarah Boston and Jill Louw, *Disorderly Breasts* (Camden Press, 1987).

Stephen Fulder, *How to Survive Medical Treatment: a holistic approach to the risks and side-effects of orthodox medicine* (Century Paperbacks, 1987).

Rosetta Reitz, *Menopause: A positive approach* (Unwin Paperbacks, 1985).

Chemotherapy — your questions answered, Patient Information Series Number One, The Royal Marsden Hospital, 1986.

CHAPTER SEVENTEEN
Traditional and complementary treatments for breast cancer

Throughout this book, emphasis has been placed on women having choices in the way they are treated. The book has also stressed the importance of a holistic or whole-person approach to health to ensure that *all* our health needs are met. Chapter 7 looked at different approaches to health and disease and suggested that health systems based on traditional and holistic principles may have something to offer us. Chapter 10 described some of the traditional and complementary therapies available in this country. This chapter looks at a number of traditional and complementary treatments for breast cancer.

It is illegal in Britain to make public claims of curing cancer. No reputable alternative practitioner would make such a claim. But many know from their experience that alternative therapies can help in the treatment and control of the disease. Some women who have used alternative medicine seem to have made a complete recovery. Medical scientists would tend to argue that these women have had spontaneous remission or some mistake was made about their diagnosis in the first place. But thousands of women believe they have benefited and are still benefiting from traditional and complementary treatments.

One chapter cannot hope to do justice to the many traditional and complementary approaches to the treatment of breast cancer. What it can do is provide some basic information and suggestions on how to proceed if you wish to find out more.

Treatments which involve changes in diet

Diet is central to most traditional and complementary treatments for cancer. A traditional Chinese practitioner, a medical herbalist or a homoeopath would all be interested in what you eat and would probably make suggestions about changing your diet.

Penny Brohn in her book about the therapies used at the Bristol Cancer Help centre (see Further reading, page 158) suggests these guidelines:

● Reduce protein intake in general and animal protein in particular
● Reduce levels of fat
● Eat as much natural food as possible
● Eat as much raw food as possible
● Avoid salt
● Avoid sugar
● Avoid stimulants (tea, coffee, etc.)
● Think positively about what you are eating.

These guidelines are intended to help you eat a highly nourishing diet without overloading the digestive system. Naturopathic diets aim to nourish you and enhance your immune system without putting any strain on your body systems through overeating, stimulants and poisons. (Some additives and preservatives are poisonous and so is alcohol in large amounts.) Most diets start with a 'cleansing period' which may be a stricter version of a longer-term diet. This is aimed at clearing out any poisons which have built up in the body, particularly in the liver. Most people find a cleansing diet helpful and feel better for it.

Each alternative therapy will have slightly different guidelines on diet, and will combine suggestions about diet with a number of other treatments (see Chapter 10). Some modern nutritionists have argued that changes in diet can successfully treat different diseases including cancer. The most famous of these is Dr Max Gerson who developed a dietary regime which has had some success in treating cancer (see Further reading, page 158). The problem is that the treatment is exacting, expensive and lengthy. It means organizing your life around your treatment and transforming your home into a treatment unit. Beata Bishop has written about her experience of the Gerson diet and her cure of malignant melanoma (see Further reading, page 158).

For most people changing your diet is no easy matter. Organizing a healthy diet takes time and effort and some women feel they haven't got either. Money can also be a problem. Sticking to a healthy diet can be very difficult, particularly if you have an unsympathetic family who think a wholefood diet is silly. Then there's the question of which diet to choose, as some of them seem to contradict each other. Some women embark on a strict healthy diet only to find that they can't keep it up. So it's worth thinking out carefully what you *can* achieve. It's better to succeed with a few changes than to fail because you're trying to do too much at once. Here are some suggestions which may help you to overcome some of the difficulties:

● Get advice and information so that you choose a diet which seems most appropriate for *you* and that you think you will be able to keep to. See the list of useful addresses at the end of the book for cancer help centres and other centres for nutritional advice. Rather than chopping and changing, choose one diet and try to stick to that. A healthy diet is only one part of your whole-person programme. It's important not to worry too much about it

● Make sure any diet regime is explained to you so that it is clear why you are giving up some foods and not others. Understanding the diet will make it easier to stick to and easier to explain to family, friends and doctors

● Discuss any diet with other members of your household, and try to get their co-operation. It is much more difficult to change your diet without support from other people. If your household is willing to change their diet with you, all the better. They will feel the benefit of it too. If they won't change, try and get them to promise to encourage you and give you moral support

● Work out what your diet will mean in terms of additional costs. Buying seasonal fruit and vegetables won't be expensive but organically grown vegetables may be. Growing your own vegetables is a possibility. If you haven't got a garden or only have a small one, you could put your name down for an allotment. Members of your household or perhaps a group of friends could help you run it. If you know someone with an allotment who grows organically they may be happy to give you surplus fruit and vegetables or sell them to you cheap. If you need to rely on shop fruit and vegetables, wash them thoroughly as there may be chemicals on the skin or outer layers

● Check out any equipment you may need. Some diets include freshly squeezed vegetable and fruit juices. For this you will need a juicing machine. Aluminium pans kill important nutrients in food so look out for stainless steel, enamel or Pyrex pans. You may only be able to get these over a period of time but perhaps your friends could club together for a birthday present. Some women have held a fund-raising party to meet the cost

● Plan out your diet for a week in advance. This helps to avoid the temptation of breaking it. It also allows you to make it as varied as possible. It's worth getting a note-book and writing down any recipes you come across from other people's cook books or from library books. Ask your friends to look out for tasty salads and vegetarian dishes which you can try (see Further reading)

● Explain your diet to any friends and relatives so they take it seriously if you go round for a meal. In recent years people have become far more conscious of the need for a healthy diet and most will respect you for taking your diet seriously

● Most important of all, don't let the diet you choose get you down. If you feel it's too difficult to change your diet all at once, try changing one thing at a time. If you need to have a 'treat', have one and enjoy it. It's important not to feel that you're denying yourself food, particularly if eating is one of your pleasures.

Going on a special diet is a choice which some women will take and others won't. Food is an important comforter for many women and altering their diet may cause anxiety and distress. Understandably, some women will prefer not to change their diet and will look to other ways of healing themselves.

Dietary supplements

Some naturopaths will only recommend natural foods in treating cancer but others, including dietary therapists, will recommend vitamin and mineral supplements. The major source of vitamins and minerals is found in food and a well-balanced diet with a good amount of raw fruit and vegetables goes a long way towards providing necessary vitamins and minerals. The ability to use or store vitamins will vary in each person. This ability is affected by stress *and* by radiotherapy and chemotherapy (see Chapters 14 and 16).

Scientists now recognize that vitamin A deficiency can increase the likelihood of cancer. This is because vitamin A is associated with cell duplication so lack of it appears to make it easier for cells to duplicate themselves incorrectly. They also know that certain substances which are present in food, called free radicals, easily damage DNA. Other substances called anti-oxidants are very effective at mopping up these free radicals before they can cause any damage. The three best natural anti-oxidants are beta-carotene (related to vitamin A and found in carrots and most green leafy vegetables), vitamin E (present in wholemeal bread and cereals, vegetable oils, eggs and fish) and the mineral selenium (found in brewer's yeast, wholewheat, mushrooms, liver, sea foods and asparagus).

Other vitamins and minerals which are thought to be particularly helpful are:

● Vitamin C (contained in fruit and vegetables). This stimulates the production of white blood cells which are an important part of the immune system

● Vitamin B complex, a group of vitamins which help in food digestion and the production of red and white blood cells

● Zinc, magnesium and potassium, all of which help to strengthen the immune system.

Your doctor may be able to help you to work out a combination of vitamin supplements to suit your needs. She will need to take a blood sample to test for any deficiencies. This will then be sent away for a laboratory analysis. If your doctor is not familiar with this procedure, it may be simpler to contact a laboratory which specializes in this service (see addresses on page 194). They will send you any equipment you need for the blood test and make recommendations about any supplements when they have analysed the blood sample.

Some doctors and scientists, including Nobel prize winner, Linus Pauling, recommend large doses (or megadoses) of vitamins, particularly vitamin C, in the treatment of cancer. One trial showed a marked improvement in cancer patients given large amounts of ascorbic acid (vitamin C) and other cases have been documented where megadoses of vitamins have not only improved the condition but have also cured the disease.

Vitamin supplements are expensive to buy over the counter, but you can get them through your doctor on prescription. Not all doctors are clear about this so you may need to persevere. The Bristol Cancer Help Centre has clarified the situation and obtained written confirmation from the DHSS Prescription Pricing Authority in Newcastle-upon-Tyne that vitamin and mineral supplements can be ordered on the NHS and passed for payment by them. The Bristol Cancer Help Centre will provide you with this information for your GP if necessary (see Useful addresses, page 195).

Vitamin and mineral supplements won't produce miracle cures

for breast cancer but they can improve your health and contribute to controlling the disease.

Vitamin E and breast cancer

Some books suggest that Vitamin E is bad for you if you have breast cancer. This is because vitamin E appears to improve the mobility of sperm in men and lessen the possibility of miscarriage in women. It is suggested that vitamin E effects hormone activity and therefore may influence the growth of breast cancer but there is no evidence that this is the case. Vitamin E is an important vitamin in the process of healing the body. If you are at all worried about using it, seek advice from a nutritionist.

Natural remedies

All traditional systems of medicines as well as several complementary approaches use a wide range of natural products in treatment. The majority of these come from herbs and plants but there are also some mineral and animal extracts. In the case of homoeopathy, these are prepared in diluted form using homoeopathic methods.

If you are considering a traditional or complementary treatment, it is important to consult a fully qualified practitioner. Different remedies are used to treat cancer itself and to protect your immune system during treatment. Some well known remedies are described below.

Iscador This is an anthroposophic remedy extracted from mistletoe. Iscador enhances the immune response and inhibits cancer growth. In one study by Dr Rita Leroi, iscador was found to lengthen life in women with advanced breast cancer. It has also been used as a follow-up treatment for primary breast cancer.

Iscador can be taken by mouth or given by injection. Anthroposophic doctors and some homoeopathic practitioners can assess what dose you need and they can contact your own GP with instructions about how to use the drug. Your GP can then prescribe iscador on the NHS. It is usually taken every other day and many patients learn to inject themselves. A possible side-effect is a slightly increased temperature in women. This is seen as positive as it indicates an immune response.

Iscador is regularly used in the Royal Homoeopathic Hospital in Great Ormond Street in London and in other NHS homoeopathic hospitals in the country (see page 194 for list of homoeo-pathic hospitals in Britain).

Amygdalin This is also known as laetrile or B_{17}. Amygdalin is extracted from the pips and kernels of apples, apricots, grapes, peaches, plums and other fruit and some grains. Amygdalin includes a cyanide molecule in its make-up which acts on cancer cells. Some doctors and alternative practitioners are enthusiastic about its contribution to the treatment of cancer patients.

But amygdalin has its critics. They argue that amygdalin can be dangerous if improperly prescribed. It has caused heated debates and is now illegal in some states of America even though there are well-documented cases of its use in the treatment of cancer. It is not available on the NHS. More information about how to obtain amygdalin and how to use it can be obtained from the organizations listed on page 195.

Coffee and herb enemas An enema is a method of clearing the bowels of their contents. Many women will experience having an enema when they go into hospital to have a baby. Therapeutic enemas are not the same (they are sometimes called implants). The Gerson diet uses regular coffee enemas to stimulate the liver and flush out any toxic substances from the body (in other regimes herbal enemas may be used). This is done by using a gravity feed enema kit which you can use for yourself. The liquid from ground coffee or a mixture of herbs is introduced into the rectum and held in the bowels for as long as is comfortable. You then evacuate it by going to the toilet. A gravity feed enema kit can be obtained from most chemists.

Dr Bach's flower remedies These are based on the investigations of Dr Edward Bach who believed that physical illnesses are caused by mental and emotional states. During years of experimentation, he developed a selection of flower essences which are recommended for treating states of shock, feelings of despair, fear, and other emotional states. The Bach Flower Centre provides a list of essences and explains how to use them.

Ask the practitioner to explain any remedy she prescribes for you. What may appear to be strange or outlandish can have a clear and sensible explanation and this helps when you start explaining your treatment to disbelieving others. You'll find more information in Chapters 13, 14 and 16 on remedies which help to lessen the side-effects of modern treatments.

Acupuncture and acupressure

According to Chinese traditional medicine, energy or life-force flows along a network of energy pathways (meridians) in the body. When these pathways become blocked or sluggish, symptoms of ill-health appear. Acupuncture and acupressure use these meridian lines to try to revitalize and redirect the energy flow. In acupuncture, fine needles made of copper, silver or gold are inserted at special points along a particular meridian. In acupressure, the practitioner uses her fingers and hand to exert pressure along the meridian lines. In each case, the aim is to regulate energy flow.

Medical scientists have not yet discovered how acupuncture works, although it is thought that there are some similarities between meridian pathways and nerve endings linked to the nervous system. Acupuncture and acupressure are recognized by many mainstream doctors as helpful treatments for pain. Traditional acupuncture and acupressure are normally combined with other treatments such as diet and herbal remedies in the treatment of major diseases including cancer.

Exercise

Exercise may appear to have little to do with cancer but it does contribute to a whole-person treatment programme. It forms part of all traditional health systems. Yoga exercises or traditional Chinese exercises (T'ai Chi Ch'uan) are two examples of whole-person exercise which may be run as an evening class and which can be practised in your own home. Other activities like swimming, walking and cycling will help to stimulate your circulation and tone up body tissue.

It's a good idea to map out an exercise programme over a period of time. If you're out of condition, try a short walk each day to begin with and gradually build up your strength. Regular exercise can relieve stress and anxiety. It can also help to improve your health and sense of well-being.

Relaxation and breathing exercises

Relaxation is an important part of traditional and complementary treatments because it is seen as the basis on which a mind/body healing process can begin. Most people associate relaxation with putting your feet up and nodding off. But there's more to relaxation than that. It means consciously relaxing the different parts of the body, clearing the mind of the clutter of everyday life, and experiencing moments of peacefulness and rest in body and mind. It is this deep resting of the 'inner self' as well as the body which has been part of traditional medicine for thousands of years.

Most people have to *learn* to relax fully. Some women will find it difficult to make the time to leave everything and relax for a quarter of an hour. The first thing is to find a quiet, warm place to relax. Relaxation is best done lying on your back on a firm surface (floor ideally) with a folded blanket or small pillow to support your head. You can lie with your knees bent and your feet flat on the floor or resting on a chair — this helps relax the lower back to the ground. If you lie straight then keep your heels together and let your toes fall apart. Have your arms slightly out to your sides, palms upwards or rest your palms on your belly. Relax your shoulders.

It may not be possible for you to lie on the floor. You can relax in bed or sitting on a chair. The main thing is to make sure your body is evenly and fully supported and that you are warm enough. Don't curl on your side or lie on your front as this will prevent you breathing well.

Some women find playing a tape helpful while they're learning to relax. You may like to put this exercise on tape to help you begin relaxation.

● Once you are in position, close your eyes and feel your body beginning to relax. Let the full weight of your body sink back to your support

● Direct your thoughts to each part of your body in turn, to the muscles and the joints. Let your legs become heavy and relaxed, letting go of any tension as you breath out. Let both your feet, your toes, your ankles, knees and thighs become soft and heavy. Now do the same with your arms, relaxing your hands, fingers, wrists, elbows and pay particular attention to dropping your shoulders back and down

● Think now about your back and your spine, let any tension drain away. Each time you breathe out, let your back spread and relax, more and more. Feel as if the breath is coming in through the pores of the skin on the back, filling your whole back from the buttocks to the neck and shoulders and that as you breathe out your whole back eases back and rests completely. Relax the pelvis and the waist. Don't hold the stomach muscles in, allow your stomach to feel soft and quiet

● Let go of any tension on your neck and throat. The chin should tuck slightly down towards your chest. Don't throw your head back. Let the full weight of your head be supported. Your eyes should be completely closed and the face soft. Let all the muscles in your face and around your skull relax so that the skin feels smooth and not tight. Your mouth is closed, your lips lightly touching, your tongue rests behind your lower teeth

● As your body becomes quiet and your eyes still, your brain begins to relax and your breathing becomes steadier. Continue the process of relaxing your body, letting go as you breathe out, allowing each part of you to become soft, heavy and open. Pay particular attention to areas which feel tense or painful

● Be aware of breathing in and out evenly. You may wish to count, say to four, as you breathe in and as you breathe out. Never force the breath. Gradually let your breath out become a little longer and deeper. Feel as if all the physical and mental tension is eased away as the breath leaves your body. Each breath in brings new life and healing, each breath out takes the toxins and the tensions with it. Continue in this pattern of breathing for a few minutes — normal breathing in, full deep breath out. Relax more and more

● When you are ready gradually bring your breathing back to normal. Continue slow gentle breathing for a few moments. Become aware of the room around you. Stretch a little. Open your eyes slowly. If you're lying down, turn on your side before you get up.

If you decide to put this on tape, read it slowly, pausing after each sentence or ask a friend to prepare this for you together with some soothing music which you can listen to while you relax. You can obtain ready made tapes from the Bristol Cancer Help Centre, The British Holistic Medical Association and the Matthew Manning Centre (see pages 193-5). When you have gained some experience in relaxation, you can use it in other areas of your life: before you go to sleep, on your way to work, or in hospital outpatients using a shortened version.

Visualization or mental imagery and meditation

Most traditional and complementary practitioners believe the powers of the mind play an important role in healing ourselves.

Mental imagery is one way of developing our own self-healing abilities. While you are relaxing, you can imagine to yourself a visual image of the process of healing taking place in your body.

People choose different images. Some women may need the help of a counsellor or therapist to choose a meaningful one for them. As we saw in Chapters 14 and 16, visualization can also be used during radiotherapy and chemotherapy.

Mental imagery can be used to help you relax fully. For example, while you're relaxing, think of yourself in a beautiful place, a sunny garden with flowers and birds. You can hear the hum of bees and other insects. Imagine the sun warming your limbs, relaxing your body and giving you a sense of well-being. Many women find that with practice, they can use visualization easily and get great comfort from it.

Meditation is taking this process one step further, allowing your mind to rest quietly, aware of your breathing, reaching a stillness in which to experience healing in body and mind. It may help to use words like 'I am healing myself' or 'All is well' or concentrate on feelings of well-being. If you feel your life is full of anxiety and pain, these times of relaxation and meditation can help you to find moments of peace and wholeness, and help to renew your courage and energy at difficult times.

Healing

Healing can be done in different ways. Some healers see their skills as revitalizing the healing energy within each individual. Others see themselves as passing on their healing energy to the person who is ill and yet others see their role as creating a pathway for divine intervention.

Some healers use meditation or prayer as a medium for healing and others prefer physical contact, using their hands to heal. Some women find that a healer provides a certain wisdom and quality of support that no other health worker can give. Most healers give their services free because they wish to share this special ability to help others.

Other treatment choices — where to find out more

These brief notes on traditional and complementary therapies leave many gaps. Some other alternative and complementary treatments are described in earlier chapters in reducing the side-effects of modern treatments. Others are discussed in relation to living with cancer, for example the role of counsellors, psychologists and psychotherapists (see Chapter 19). More information about all these and other traditional and complementary treatments for breast cancer can be obtained from the reading list at the end of the chapter and from the organizations listed on page 192.

No traditional and complementary treatments claim miracle cures for breast cancer. What they do claim is that by using treatments which assist our body's own resources and healing powers we give ourselves the best opportunity to regain good health in body and in mind.

Further reading

Beata Bishop, *A Time to Heal* (Severn House Publishers, 1985). This book describes Ms Bishop's recovery and cure of malignant melanoma using the Gerson therapy.

Penny Brohn, *The Bristol Programme: An introduction to the holistic therapies practised by the Bristol Cancer Help Centre* (Century Paperbacks, 1987).

Ian Gawler, *You Can Conquer Cancer: The self-help guide to the way back to health* (Thorsons, 1986).

Shirley Harrison, *New Approaches to Cancer: What everyone needs to know about orthodox and complementary methods for prevention, treatment and cure* (Century Paperbacks, 1987).

Kit Mouat, *Fighting for Our Lives: An introduction to living with cancer* (Heretic Books, 1984). This book gives a brief outline of different treatments for cancer including traditional and complementary approaches.

CHAPTER EIGHTEEN

Making choices about treatment

Making choices about treatment is a complicated process. Decisions are often made under stress and without enough information. We each have to make our own choices about our health, because what works for one woman may not help another.

The important thing is to work out what suits you best. There are many sources of information: national bodies like the Breast Care and Mastectomy Association, BACUP and Cancerlink; your consultant who can discuss with you your preferences and answer your questions; perhaps above all the experience of other women is an invaluable source of knowledge. In this chapter six women recount, in their own words, their experience of trying to make their own choices.

Chris

Actually it was my husband who found the lump. It was hard and round and it felt fixed, not movable. I was in the middle of a period and thought I'd leave it to see if it went down. In the end I went to my doctor with a sore throat and I told him that I'd got this lump in my breast. He said he wasn't terribly worried about it, but made an appointment for me to see a consultant a fortnight later.

Chris was given a needle biopsy and asked to return the following week for the results. The consultant told her he thought it was a fibrous lump of some kind which would have to be removed.

I came away and immediately started to panic. I felt ill. From one day to the next I lived in a dream world that week. I gathered all the information I could and ran round like an idiot. But I felt much happier doing it because I was doing something constructive towards it rather than sitting down and thinking, 'Oh dear, I've got breast cancer, wherever will it end?' On the Wednesday when I went back he sent me for a mammogram so when I got home I read up about mammograms.

At her next appointment the consultant told Chris he would like to do a lumpectomy.

Then he stood back from me towards the students in the room and said, 'How would you feel if we have to do a mastectomy whilst you're under the anaesthetic?' I said, 'You're joking. This is a lump, I want you to tell me what the lump is.' He made me afraid then, I thought, 'Why is he saying this without knowing what it is?' I was on my own, I didn't go with anyone because if I do have to stand up to a crisis, I can face it better alone. I wanted to be strong and while you're on your own you're strong. So I thought, 'Right, get as much information from him as you can.' I said, 'Why are you saying this? This is some sort of fibrous lump.' He said, 'Yes it is, and all lumps have to be removed.' So I said, 'I suppose I have to rely on your judgement,' and left it at that.

Chris asked her GP if it was worth getting a second opinion but he thought not. When she went into hospital a week later, the consultant came to see her and explained he wanted to do a wide lumpectomy. He mentioned the possibility of radiotherapy.

I said 'Oh no. Hang on a minute. You're taking the lump away. . .Come back and we'll discuss it when I've had a chance to look into what radiotherapy does. I know nothing about it and I'm not sure I want it.' he said, 'Fine, OK we'll do that.'

Chris was allowed home soon after the operation.

I thought, 'Oh great, it's just been a fibrous lump that they've been able to take away.'

She met the mastectomy nurse just before she left.

On the third day after leaving hospital the mastectomy nurse rang me and asked if I could pop in and see her. I didn't for one minute think there was any sinister reason behind this. As a matter of luck my husband offered to run me up. I'm so glad he was with me because when we got there she said the consultant wanted a word. . .and that's when the bombshell dropped. He said, 'The results of your test have come back and they are positive.' I said, 'How do you mean "positive"?' He said, 'It is cancerous.' He said, 'By doing a sub-cutaneous mastectomy we can save the outside of your skin and we won't have to do any other treatment, because I know you feel a bit unsure about radiotherapy. Let me put it to you that you have a very good chance of survival.'

I suddenly thought 'Oh dear, why is he talking about survival?' It just didn't sink in. It was quite horrific.

Because it was just before Christmas and there was a vacant bed, Chris had to choose between going in that night or waiting until after the holiday. At first she was reluctant to go in straight away.

When we got home I decided I would go back. I sort of thought 'Well, he's answered all the questions I wanted to ask and I feel he's been quite fair.' So I went back that night and the morning after he did the operation.

Whether or not it was a bit too quick I'm still wondering. I still have doubts that maybe I would have been better asking someone else's opinion, going somewhere else and saying 'Look can you save the breast?. . .'The thing that was worrying me was the radiotherapy because I know it can disfigure your breast anyway. . .I thought, 'I've got enough to handle, I can't handle having radiotherapy as well.'

The subcutaneous mastectomy left Chris's nipple intact but the consultant wasn't sure it would establish its own blood supply.

The district nurse came and she was wonderful. . .she brought me the *BACUP News*, introduced me to things like that to get my morale up. She told me about vitamins. J. brought me that lovely book *A Gentle Way with Cancer* and I read up on how to keep myself healthy and about nourishing foods and I thought, 'This is not going to happen again' I sort of delved into that then . . . I started to feel quite good about it. Positive. I suppose that's the word they use in hospital as well. I'm not saying there weren't down days but during the time of the district nurse coming, her helping to clean it for me using usol and paraffin. . .They really looked after me. My sister in law is a district nurse and she brought me these lovely dressings — a kind of gauze with honey and glycerine to keep the nipple moist and feed it. It's almost as if it's given a skin graft because new skin pushed itself up and it survived. At the same time I was taking vitamins and still do. I went back four weeks later and he said, 'You really have looked after this haven't you?'

Chris was offered a prosthesis.

> Now that was traumatic. I hated it. . .odd sensations and I could not imagine myself wearing that thing inside my bra for the rest of my life. But I didn't feel downhearted about it. It was almost like having a new toy. I'd got this shoe box under my arm and I thought, 'I've got this new toy, I'll try it on when I get home!' It felt all right. It didn't cause any problems on the outside but inwardly I hated it. I just thought, ' I can't be doing with this thing. It's annoying me, it's not me. It's not feminine and it's not what I want to be.' So eventually I started to go round the house without the prosthesis in. It felt better for that and it felt kind of nice and comforting to put your hand in and feel your warm flesh and not a plastic thing.

About six months later Chris was offered an implant, to which she agreed. She reflects on the decision.

> Now looking back on it, I think it was too soon. I would say to any woman who is considering having breast re-construction — give yourself some time to get to like your-self as you are as a one-breasted woman. Get to love the person you see in the mirror. Get your husband to love the person. That is something I've cheated myself on. I felt as though I probably haven't known the one-breasted woman long enough. Although during the six months that I knew her, I wasn't terribly happy with her. I accepted that I'd had a mastectomy. I felt fine about the operation. But the prosthe-sis — I hated the feel of it.
>
> When I went to have the permanent implant put in, it was almost as if I was reliving the mastectomy. . .It was the trauma again of leaving everybody. . .After I came round I felt terribly deflated. I thought, 'Oh dear me, it's not what I wanted, it doesn't look like I wanted it to look.' It brought home the memories of the mastectomy even more. It was kind of like, 'You've had the mastectomy, we've given you an implant, that's all we can do for you, now toddle off. We can't do any more.'
>
> I don't know if I made the right decision then. . .I felt that I'd been channelled into it. I was the right age and the right sort of mastectomy and the right type of tumour. I think he

must have looked at me and thought, 'Here's this young woman, only 31, two young children, we'll do it for her. We can rebuild her!' But I feel great now. I've coped with it . . . I feel happier. It feels nice to feel warm skin there. I'm not saying that it's any better sexually in that it can't be any more than an inward prosthesis. There's no stimulation there. It's softened down a great deal and I don't feel it's this great bulky thing sticking out on my chest any more. I feel happy about it.

I would say to other women, 'Be sure you're making the right choice. Be sure that you want this doing.' I think women need time. I think it's about time we said to surgeons, 'Hang on. I know you think you're doing the right job. But I don't want to be a number and I want some time to consider how it's going to affect me as a person'.

Jo

I'm 53 years old. My attitude to breasts was always to be proud of the size and shape of them but I was sexually repressed and therefore I hid them. I used to walk around with my shoulders hunched. And then as I got older, I ceased to think about them . . . until I got breast cancer. Then suddenly they became centre stage and then it wasn't the fear of mutilation that galvanized me but actually my knowledge of my mother's history of losing a breast, unnecessarily in my opinion.

I found a lump and went to my GP who examined the breasts. She said they were very 'nodular' — the term she used — and not to worry about it. This was joy to my ears and I promptly went off and forgot about it. But I kept feeling this lump and it was still there. But I didn't go back. It's like a game, a kind of trial. I thought 'Well, she said it was nodular, so it's all right. I'm not going to think about it.' But then I did secretly keep examining it. And then a friend of mine had breast cancer and I was telling her about this lump. She said, 'You're mad. What are you doing? It's a year since you went. Go back and tell her.' But I didn't want to see her again so my friend told me to go to a breast screening clinic which is what I did. Within three or four days I was in hospital. It was as quick as that.

I went to the breast screening clinic and saw a really nice nurse. She felt it and looked at it and I had a mammogram done. She said that it was a bit dodgy and that I'd have to go back and see a doctor. I went back the next day and a doctor did a needle biopsy.

He said I needed to go into hospital anyway because the lump ought to come out. He said by the time I got into hospital they'd know the results of the needle biopsy. I went into hospital very quickly, that day. The results hadn't come through. It was like a nightmare hanging round waiting.

The following morning a nurse suddenly appeared, put the curtains round and said, 'It's not the good news you'd hoped for'. That's all she said and I burst into tears. About half an hour later, after me sitting on the bed, howling, clutching my book on breast cancer, this group of people came round the bed. The doctor got out this board and said, 'That's the one that's coming off.' I just went berserk, I said, 'Why is it coming off?' He said he couldn't tell me as he wasn't my consultant. I asked him to tell me what the reason for the decision. He said he couldn't tell me that either as he didn't have my notes with him. I asked him who I could talk to. 'He's down in the operating theatre,' he said, 'would you sign a consent form?' I said I wouldn't sign anything yet.

I got out of bed and rang a friend who had breast cancer. She told me I didn't have to have a mastectomy, I could have a lumpectomy. People kept coming in and asking me to sign the consent form. They kept sending different nurses. I told them that unless I could see 'whoever he is' in half an hour, I was going home. All total bravado. Finally the consultant came to see me. He asked what the problem was. I told him that my mother had a mastectomy then died of liver cancer six weeks later. 'So if anything's going to be done, I want it staged. I do not want an amputation that isn't necessary.' He felt my breast and said 'Well it's quite a big lump. I think you should have a mastectomy.' I said that I didn't want that so he said 'All right then, you can have a lumpectomy,' and off he went, flapping up the ward.

I signed the consent form, had a pre-med and within half an hour I was down there. I woke up with a drip in my arm. My breast was still there, I remember thinking 'Thank God for that,' but feeling terrified. That night my period started. I bled all over the bed. I felt so embarrassed.

Two days later I left hospital. There was no counselling at all. As I went to leave I said to the nurse I hadn't been told anything about what to do. She said not to be so impatient. They were really fed up with me for making such a fuss. I hadn't been told how to change the dressing. She said, 'I'll give you a dressing and you change it in two days. Here's a thing for a bone scan and you'll have to come for a blood test and a liver scan.' I thought 'God, it's all over my body.' They don't tell you that they're just laying down information. She said, 'We'll send you a note when the results of the biopsy are through.' So I went away and went home and waited to die.

My friend arranged for a bereavement counsellor to call. She came and talked to me and stayed for hours. She was like an angel. I talked through all my worries. She said, 'You're not going to die. The fact that your mother died six weeks after. . .it's very unlikely that it would happen to you too.'

I saw a GP. All she said was 'Would you like some anti-depressants?' When I asked for a certificate, she said, 'You don't want me to put 'breast cancer' on the certificate, do you?' I asked why not and she said 'Well, you don't really want the people at work to know.' I thought, 'What is it I've entered into?' I said, 'I want to know what I've had done.' I just wanted to have the certificate. I just wanted evidence of what was happening to me. It's like you've invented a nightmare and everywhere along the line you're supposed to keep quiet, hide the fact that you're ill, take the anti-depressants.

The path for me in choosing traditional medicine was to go first of all to the Bristol Cancer Help Centre. I welcomed their regime like a new ritual in life. It kept me together. Then, when I realized it didn't seem adequate enough I went to a naturopath. The first woman worked on my back and within a week I couldn't type, because my back was so locked up as I'd never had it touched in my life.

Anyway that all settled down and I haven't had any problems. I went to the Yoga Association for a weekend on holistic health. There was a group of people discussing where resources were. Yoga seemed to me a good way to relax. I got a lot of information at the yoga weekend. I found a much more experienced naturopath who uses Indian herbs.

I saw this naturopath but my body didn't respond to what she was doing. She said, 'I don't know what else I can do really except keep doing this.' Finally. . .I found a good acupuncturist at this practice in Highgate. She said, 'We treat a lot of cancer patients here.' I thought, 'Thank God for that.' She said, 'Here's something you can read about Chinese health, so that you know a bit more about it. We can't tackle the cancer direct, but we can tackle the whole body and I can work on the breast in various ways, with moxibustion (a form of herbal heat treatment applied to acupuncture points), and other techniques.'

So that was that, I kind of gave myself to them. I didn't take any responsibility for myself but I have gradually learnt that they are not the answer to my problem. I have to monitor my own life. I can't just keep going back and saying, 'Oh God, I'm ill again,' and she saying, 'Well, have you broken your diet? Do you ever get enough sleep?' I've learnt over the last four years of going there to monitor myself much more, to have more holidays. I've done assertiveness training. I'm a totally different person. I used to be really rebellious and stroppy but that doesn't get rid of your anger. I've learnt to say what I think and people don't like it. Recently I've learnt to temper it with jokes and things like that.

David and I have a marvellous relationship and that's contributed to my health a lot. I met him at a therapy weekend. Two completely neurotic 50-year-olds sitting there. We got on well and have got very fond of each other and here we are, four years later, really very happy.

If I were asked what would be the first thing to do when told that I had breast cancer, it would either be to find out a healthy way of discharging anger, or I should go to an assertiveness training course so that I could at last begin to establish what my needs were and try and get them met.

Vera

I first discovered a lump myself during a routine self-examination 10 months ago. Having breast cancer had always been a great fear for me — my mother and grandmother died of it at an early age. I decided to wait a month to see if it went down after my period. It didn't, so I went to see my GP. She was very reassuring and said it was probably a blocked milk duct — I'd not long stopped breast feeding my daughter. 'To be on the safe side' she referred me to the breast clinic at a London teaching hospital. I saw a consultant two weeks later.

After tests, Vera was told at her second outpatients appointment that the lump was a benign cyst, and it was aspirated. Her relief was shattered a week later by a phone call from the hospital asking her to return to repeat the aspiration. The junior doctor who spoke to her would not tell her anything more. Suspicious, she felt she would rather know the truth immediately than wait in uncertainty until her next appointment. She repeatedly phoned the hospital to try and speak to someone who would give her more information, but without success.

> On my return the next week I was told straight away that cancer cells had been found in the fluid taken from the cyst. . . I still feel that I should have been told straight away, rather than the hospital keeping up what felt like a deception, which completely undermined my trust in them.
>
> The first reaction to my diagnosis was shock, my mind just went numb. That lasted for about three weeks. I felt frightened, desperate and very lonely. I was in no position to make any kind of informed decision about my treatment. I was so overwhelmed by the news of having cancer and was convinced I would anyhow be dead very soon. The issue of what treatments to choose seemed unimportant, though I desperately wanted more information about the extent of my cancer to assess my chances. Fortunately I had earlier made enquiries about my surgeon through the Community Health Council. He had a reputation for doing minimal operations so I felt vaguely reassured that I could trust his judgement.

Vera's lumpectomy revealed that the cancer had spread to the lymph nodes, and she was told she would need radiotherapy and chemotherapy to treat it.

> I resigned myself to the radiotherapy quite quickly, although that's not to say I wasn't sometimes doubtful whilst having my treatment. . . I had always thought of myself as a very tough and strong person and physical side-effects didn't worry me too much. I found coping with the discomfort after the operation almost a distraction from the thoughts about cancer and dying that preoccupied me most of the time. I badly wanted something to be done about the cancer and the hospital procedure offered some sort of reassurance. I did — and still do — feel a great dilemma between wanting to be informed and in control of decisions and on the other hand feeling that the whole thing about the cancer was too much for me to handle and wanting help.
>
> Before the cancer I had opted for alternative medicine during pregnancy and childbirth, but cancer, a life and death

issue, seemed altogether on another scale. I didn't at the time have the 'alternative' support network I have now. Friends had bombarded me with books and information about alternative therapies but it was all too new and unfamiliar and I hadn't the time or energy to get my mind round it. At that time I didn't know anybody refusing radiotherapy or orthodox treatment altogether.

As far as I could make out. . . there was a statistically proven reduced risk of recurrence when having radiotherapy following lumpectomy. The depression of the immune system seemed an acceptable risk to take. So I felt reasonably satisfied with having radiotherapy whilst following a naturopathic diet, doing visualization, relaxation, etc.

I was horrified at the idea of chemotherapy. . . terrified at the idea of toxic drugs being pumped into my body and invading me. The decision to go ahead with it was fairly agonizing. I was, and still am, sceptical about its effectiveness.

I finally agreed to it after much reading, talking to friends and also quite detailed discussions with hospital staff which I really appreciated. I did feel at the time that the hospital was my lifeline. They were the people dealing with my cancer and I needed to remain in touch with them. I liked the thought of something being done about the cancer and, I suppose, having early on resigned myself to aggressive orthodox medical treatment, it seemed logical to continue. Another aspect of all this treatment was that it temporarily made me *visibly* ill. It sounds a bit strange, but it's immensely difficult and confusing to try and deal with an illness which is at this stage *invisible*. I had just been diagnosed with cancer, a disease that might kill me, and in some way it seemed more appropriate to lie in bed and be ill. It also offered friends and family a concrete way to become involved and supportive, by helping with the housework, child care, etc.

The cancer diagnosis for me precipitated a complete life crisis, and I felt I needed to rethink all aspects of my life. . . I felt a great impatience and urgency about getting priorities right and not bothering any more with work that had bored me a lot of the time, with housework that seemed a waste of time, with relationships that felt superficial and meaningless now. In some ways the knowledge of the cancer and the threat to my life gave me strength and put me back in touch with my real needs. I had to sort out my problems and live now, or else it might be too late.

Functioning again as a 'normal' person still feels rather artificial especially since I feel the threat to my life is still acute and real. I still think about cancer every day and have patches of depression, but also times of feeling intensely alive and happy. Sticking to the Bristol diet, and the relaxation and visualization, is more of an effort now, though immediately helpful when I do it. It's certainly harder to take my needs and well-being really seriously now that there are no physical manifestations of an illness. I still see a psychiatrist at the hospital for counselling, which I find extremely helpful. It gives me time and space to concentrate on the cancer and voice my thoughts and fears. The 'unthinkable' has happened to me and it's an ongoing process learning to cope with it.

Cynthia

My choices were really in the orthodox system. I've always known about homoeopathic medicines. My grandmother used them. I had a fair knowledge of alternatives and had used them but I never really thought of it as a treatment for cancer. I was very fairly dealt with by the system. I had an excellent surgeon and all the way through he consulted me about the next step. I had ample opportunity to say what I wanted.

I've always had a thing about breast cancer, maybe because I've always had lumpy breasts, the left one in particular. This made it difficult, both psychologically and practically to feel for lumps. Consequently I used to go to my GP's well-woman clinic every year for a breast examination. I went to the doctor's because my periods started coming every two weeks and, as it was about the time of my well-woman check up, I asked him to do a routine check while I was there. He said he thought there was a lump but he wasn't sure and asked me to come back. Three weeks later he said, 'Well, I think it's OK but I would like you to see a breast surgeon.' I was given an appointment four weeks later with the consultant. He was very straight and extremely kind. He said, 'Well obviously the reason you're here is that it could be cancer. I'll arrange for you to have a mammogram on Wednesday. I'll see you next Monday. I know you're going to be screwed up until then but I'm afraid there's nothing I can do about it.'

I had the mammogram. At the next appointment he told me he strongly suspected that it was cancer and asked me to come in on Friday. He gave me the choice of a mastectomy but I opted for a lumpectomy if possible. He promised me he would only do aggressive surgery if cancer was proven. I had signed a consent form allowing the lymph glands to be removed. After I had had the operation I realized that this was what they'd done. When the results came back he advised a mastectomy because he'd found a few other tumours around the one he'd taken away.

I was very upset at the time not least because my husband had had multiple sclerosis diagnosed that very same week. It was all a bit hairy! The consultant was very good. I said, 'If you're sure this has got to be done, I'm happy to go along with it.' but he said, 'No, I'll definitely take a second opinion.' He arranged a meeting for us all. The consultant radiologist said, 'There's no doubt about it, this breast has got to go and every vestige of cancer will then be removed and the radiotherapy will just be a back-up.'

I went on Tuesday, I had the mastectomy on the Wednesday and came home on Saturday. I had no stitches because he was trying out a new technique. I'm not sure what it was. I think it was some kind of adhesive. He told me that he'd never done it before but it all healed up very well so he was very pleased about it.

Before the operation I'd discussed with him the use of homoeopathic medicine. I'd smuggled some in when I'd had the lumpectomy and he said he was very happy for me to use anything. I was extremely lucky. I had suppositories for post-operative pain. They had delayed reaction so were taken with the pre-med and they started to work as soon as the anaesthetic wore off. I had no pain after the lumpectomy. After the mastectomy I was put to sleep for about twelve hours or so and after that I didn't need painkillers for anything. I wasn't being brave, I just didn't need them. I felt my choices were really very good.

After the operation the back of my arm was quite numb but now I'm getting the feeling back again. When I had radiotherapy I peeled. They told me that the skin would be sore and might weep but it didn't. I had the sort of discomfort you get with sunburn but not anything traumatic. When it became sore and peeled I was given some cream to take home with me. The nurse said I could use it on any burns. Five months after the radiotherapy I felt some tightness in the area of the shoulder but there's no swelling as such.

I've had excellent back-up from the hospital. It's the only one of its kind in the NHS. They've got a cancer social worker. She runs a session on Friday mornings for relaxation and so forth. I haven't been because quite honestly I've had so much information flooding in I have enough to be going on with. I know what I have to do. They've had a relaxation and visualization tape produced and they encourage the use of homoeopathy and anything alternative at the hospital.

I've found meditation very helpful. I was involved with the peace movement for a very long time and I have this very strong feeling that peace has to begin inside the individual. I'm taking things gradually and I really didn't think I was going to see the spring and now I've seen the summer and beginning to think I might see next year. If you could see me you'd say that's quite ridiculous, you'd say, 'She looks the picture of health.' It's the mental coming to terms with it, I think that's most difficult.

So that's my story. It's quite difficult to have confidence in what you're doing. I have great highs and great lows really. Looking at it very subjectively, if I hadn't gone through the trauma of all this which has been one of the dreads of my life, I wouldn't have gained in other directions. Emotionally, I think I had to go through this to re-assess my life.

Peggy

I had my breast off in 1981. One morning I woke up with a very bad migrane. You know how you always think, 'Oh, I would like to be sick!' So I phoned up my boss and said, 'I can't come into work because I can't walk and I can't drive. A little later I'll take a couple of distalgesics and get my head down.' I rubbed my chest and felt down and there was a lump. It was no bigger than the end of my little finger and it moved. It didn't hurt. In 1937 my grandma had breast cancer and she died in 1945. She had a radical mastectomy and had radium treatment. Having said all that it's always at the back of your mind. Not me particularly but my mother thought she'd die of breast cancer.

Peggy's husband and daughter urged her to see her GP that night. She was referred to a consultant in the hospital where she worked. He examined the lump and asked her to come into the hospital the following week.

So I went in on Thursday. That afternoon the registrars came
round...Eventually they said they were going to take me
to theatre and I had to sign consent forms. I said, 'One thing
— if there is anything there, just see to it right away. Don't
bring me back to discuss it.' A lot of people want to know
what it is before they have anything done but I thought —
I haven't the time. Three months previously I had to put my
mother into a home with dementia and Parkinson's disease.
So you see I hadn't got the time.

The lump turned out to be cancerous. Peggy had a mastectomy
and tests were done to see if cancer had spread into the lymph
nodes. The surgeon asked Peggy after the operation if he had made
the right decision in following her instructions.

I said 'You did the right thing. Knowing me, I would have
always had a niggling doubt if you hadn't removed it all.'

When her husband and daughter came to see her they were
shocked and upset.

I told my husband, 'Your mother died of cancer and your
father died of cancer and somebody in that office has just
told you that's what they've done to me. But I'm going to
live. It's something I'll cope with provided everybody treats
me normally. I don't want to be treated like an invalid.'

Once she was home Peggy arranged to have a prosthesis fitted
as soon as possible.

I went to the hospital and was fitted up...I went home and
phoned my daughter and said 'Sandra, I can jump up and
down and I move!' And of course that's it. You can get over
these things. And really my arthritis bothers me more now.
You could let it get to you but what's the point? Cancer is
a word that people use — but people die of other things as
well.
    I came out of hospital on the Wednesday and I thought
I'll get on with my life now. Then my mother died the following Tuesday. Before I came out I asked the doctor if I could
drive my car. I said my husband had said we could buy an
automatic, but the doctor said, 'No, don't buy an automatic.
You must make that arm work.' On Sunday I told my husband I wanted to drive my car but he said no. His friend
came round and I asked him. His friend said he'd take me
down the motorway because D. was nervous. So in just over
a week of the op, I was driving down the motorway — and

it was a good job I did with my mother dying on the Tuesday. I was an only daughter and had all the running about to do. I just had to get in that car and drive and get myself sorted out.

Peggy went back to work after a holiday in Tunisia and has had no recurrence of cancer. She joined the Mastectomy Support Group at her hospital.

There doesn't appear to be a way for people to get to know each other at this end of the city. It's a great pity. . . I'm told counselling should be done after the mastectomy. Personally I think that a bit of hope goes a long way before. . . My GPs call on me from time to time to go and jump up and down and talk to women who are having mastectomies and aren't happy about it.

Having a prosthesis can have its funnier side.

In 1983 I went to Portugal for my holidays, lovely beaches but of course it is the Atlantic. Big rollers. There I was on the beach in the water when all of a sudden a big wave came over — twenty feet high and it took me down to the sea bed like a cork and up I bobbed. I thought, 'Oh my God, I've lost my boob', and I had. After the tide changed my husband and his friend went to the beach to look for it — to see if it had been washed up. The following morning they went down again but no luck. These things are expensive — in the region of £50 and I said if I've got to pay for it again I want it from the insurance company. But I had to report the loss!

Peggy suffers from osteoarthritis which gives her a lot of pain. She has had radioactive injections for her knees.

I live every day as it comes. OK, I get arthritis in my shoulders and the small of my back and in my neck and it all takes little turns now and again and it drives me nuts. Cancer is a treatable and curable thing but there's no cure for arthritis yet. Coping with cancer is really mind over matter but the arthritis is an ongoing thing. It bothers me but I put up with it.

I always say nobody knows what they are going to die of or when. What's the use of me getting uptight. I might get cancer again — I might not. I might get run over by a bus.

When I went to be fitted for a new prosthesis I saw a lady

I used to meet when I took my daughter to school. She turned out to have had a mastectomy six years ago — a year before mine. I said, 'But I've seen you in the last six years — you've never mentioned it' She said, 'I don't discuss it.' I said 'Why not?' She said, 'Well why do you feel it's necessary to discuss it?' I said, 'Well I look at it this way — here am I five years on. Still here, fairly fit and very active — it has got to give somebody hope.'

Margaret

A routine cervical smear test and breast check-up at my GP's clinic revealed a small lump in the underside of the left breast, My GP immediately referred me to the breast clinic at the local hospital and I saw the consultant there three days later. I was impressed and reassured by the speed with which my GP referred me and by the thoroughness of the examination and tests. In retrospect, I'm unhappy about the delay in the follow-up and the eventual decision to operate.

The results of Margaret's first examination and tests were negative and on her next visit three months later, there was no increase in the size of the lump. At her next three months check-up the lump seemed to have enlarged and she was advised to have it removed.

I suppose I should have guessed from the speed with which a hospital bed was arranged, that the surgeon was not entirely convinced by the test results and was suspicious about the lump — which he later admitted — but I was happy to take the results at face value, I suppose because that was what I wanted to hear.

In hospital Margaret was visited by the consultant and his team who explained what was proposed — the removal of the lump and a frozen section biopsy with the possibility of removal of the lymph glands in the armpit followed by radiotherapy if cancer was evident.

There could be no question of a patient being unaware of what was to be done. There was no compulsion to accept what was offered — but there was no consideration of alternatives, it was the established procedure or nothing. Actually, I was quite willing to accept the treatment offered as I was relieved that the consultant hadn't recommended a mastectomy, which is, I believe, still the standard practice in many hospitals. At that time I was unaware of any holistic treatments for cancer, but have since read Penny Brohn's book on the Bristol Programme with great interest.

The lump proved to be cancerous so Margaret had lymph nodes removed as well. After the operation she was visited by a physiotherapist who gave her arm exercises to do.

> We were also visited by a young woman from the support clinic who had had a mastectomy seven years before and looked radiantly healthy and fit. She was very encouraging. Another woman from the support clinic came to talk about a prosthesis and showed me a sample. My reaction was illogical and over-emotional. I found the thing quite repellant, like a piece of raw veal, and I was quite frank about how disgusting I found it. The poor woman was very taken aback. But I felt adamant that if 'me' from now on was a person with a lop-sided figure, that was the way it would be. Actually, the difference in size and shape is not terribly noticeable and I'm unaware of it most of the time.

Soon after Margaret's return home radiotherapy treatment started.

> My first appointment was for examination, routine tests and 'planning'. I didn't know what this would involve. My husband took a day off so that he could be with me, for which I was heartily thankful. The routine tests were uneventful but took quite a time, with visits to various departments. I found the 'planning' session quite gruelling though. It involved lying flat on my back with arms up, holding a padded section of 'broomhandle' across my forehead and keeping as still as possible while the radiologists worked out the exact placing and direction for the radiotherapy machine. It was the only time in my entire treatment that I felt like a clinical object...feeling like a tiny cog in some high-tech machine whose workings were totally beyond me. The actual treatment began a week later and went on daily for just over six weeks. It became rather like a club — one always met the same people, and chatted and had coffee together while waiting.
> When the treatment finished there was once more a sense of being a little at a loss to be back in the 'real' world, on one's own. I was very run-down and weak, partly from inactivity but largely, I think, from sustained stress. Walking 100

yards to the shops and back was something of an ordeal at first and I could cope with nothing energetic. I also felt very depressed and haunted by a sense that maybe I was living on borrowed time. Friends and family were very supportive, though the efforts of one or two were counter-productive and one or two revealed their own dread by being quite unable to refer to cancer either by name or at all, by completely ignoring the fact that I had been ill in any way. My husband Ron was my best support — very comforting when needed, but he also has an aggressive, even black, sense of humour which was invaluable in making me see the farcical elements in otherwise grim situations.

Eventually I came to see that I was in danger of boring myself to death — and probably those around me too! — and I decided to drive myself into a more positive course. I increased the amount of fresh fruit and vegetables in our meals, cutting out meat entirely (my husband is very tolerant of 'being done good to' and happily eats this diet too). I also take a multi-vitamin supplement daily, do deep breathing exercises in the garden each morning and try to spend a part of each day outside. I do a ten-minute sequence of exercises each morning, nothing taxing but it tones up the muscles and improves breathing and circulation.

Margaret also fits in a variety of other activities.

Medau movement class, croquet, hill-walking and cycling. I practise relaxation in the form of autogenic training. I've found it extremely helpful, not only in improving my health, but also in coping with other stress factors. My general health is better now than it has been for years, I sleep well and suffer less from fatigue.

A number of women have written about their experience of breast cancer. Several books are listed at the end of Chapter 19.

CHAPTER NINETEEN

Living with breast cancer

This chapter looks at some of the problems in adjusting to living with breast cancer. It looks at the difficulties in coming to terms with a life threatening disease and the anguish many women feel about their altered body appearance. It suggests ways you can seek help and ways in which you can help yourself in overcoming these problems.

There isn't enough space in this book to explore fully the process of learning to live with cancer. Each woman will have her own way of recovering and renewing her life. Listening to other women's experiences will be particularly helpful for some women (see Further reading, page 184).

Not all women are lucky enough to remain cancer-free for the rest of their lives. This chapter looks at different treatments for secondary cancers and points out that the disease can often be successfully controlled for a number of years. There are some cases where secondary cancers have disappeared along with all other trace of cancer in the body.

Adjusting to the situation

For most women, the discovery of breast cancer is soon followed by hospital treatment. Sometimes, it is only on leaving hospital and going home that they feel the full impact of what has happened. For some of us, this can be a time of deep depression and distress which may be difficult to share with those we love. The lost certainty of good health and long life takes time to come to terms with. Your family and friends may not understand your feelings of anger and despair, particularly if you've recovered well from treatment. It may need professional help to provide the space in which to think through the meaning of this crisis in your life.

Counsellors, clinical psychologists and psychotherapists have experience of helping women in this situation and many other health workers have skills which may help you — a district nurse, or a medical social worker who has gained experience of counselling or even a bereavement counsellor. Anti-depressants can help you live through each day and keep up the appearances of coping but you may need other support to help 'heal' your worries and fears about having cancer.

Unfortunately this kind of help is not always available on the NHS. If this is the case, there are a number of independent and voluntary bodies who give counselling and support. These may be local organizations or part of a national network (see page 195). There are also therapists and counsellors who practise privately, some of whom will have a reduced scale of charges for women on low incomes.

While most counsellors and therapists won't have specialist training in supporting cancer patients, they will be able to suggest practical ways to help you renew your life. This may mean learning to relax or use mental imagery. It may mean helping you make changes in your life. All trained practitioners will have skills to listen to your feelings and anxieties and help you through this time.

> A counsellor is really like a big sister, I think. I was lucky from the very beginning. I thought I was going mad. Then someone mentioned to me about the Family Welfare Association and I got myself on their books. I got a very strait-laced woman, but she was very, very good. She listened and she reflected back. She wasn't afraid to hear me talk about dying or being afraid of what was going to happen. She seemed very stern but she did reflect back which is what I wanted to hear: that I did have some strength.

In most cities and towns there are now self-help cancer support groups (see addresses on page 195). Many women feel most at ease in such a group where talking about cancer, about experiences and about fears can be shared with other women who have the disease.

> I went to a support group very nearby every week and it was just fantastic. It really boosted me up. We had healing there and we just discussed how we were feeling and it's amazing: we were upwards of 30 or more people going to this because it was really popular.

Some women prefer to work out their own feelings about their illness on the own. They prefer to use their own resources to consider their life situation and will find an understanding through solitude and meditation. Other women will want to turn their back on the experience and get on with living.

> I was told about support groups but felt I didn't want to become involved in one — I wanted to put the experience behind me and get on with living, and it seemed that joining a support group would keep me in the role of the cancer victim.

Partners and friends need to recognize the importance of this time for adjustment and try not to ride rough-shod over our preoccupations and concerns. Comments like 'Pull yourself together', or 'Aren't you lucky that they caught it in time', don't always help and can make us feel worse. Some partners will need help themselves before they are able to give their loved ones the support they need. They too will be shocked and worried and need time to come to terms with a changed situation.

> I wish they could have counselled my husband more. The breast care nurse said something to him once when he was in the room. She made very light of it. He's not as emotional as I am and for him it was a clear-cut physical thing. But I wish she could have explained to him how I would react when I got home, that this was quite a normal reaction. He kept saying, 'I've heard enough about it, please don't go on any more. It's as hard for me as it is for you.'

If you are able to, try to talk openly to those close to you about your feelings as you go through this time of readjustment. Many people simply don't know how to talk to someone who has cancer, but if you feel able to talk about it, they will take their lead from you. If you find it very difficult to talk about it to your loved ones, and many women do, think about asking your GP or another sympathetic professional to talk to them, either with you, or for you. If your partner or family find your illness difficult to accept and discuss with you, try and get them to talk to a trained counsellor.

It is important to use the resources of trained professionals and of the cancer self-help movement, if you need to, to work through fears and feelings about cancer so they don't become a block to recovery and good health.

Coming to terms with breast surgery

The loss of a breast can lead to a deep anxiety and grief. For many women it seems as if their sexuality has been stripped from them. Your partner's sensitivity will play an important part in healing this psychological wound and you will need to recover confidence in yourself and your physical appearance.

Learning to accept yourself as a one-breasted woman and learning to explore afresh sexual enjoyment with your partner will take time. Your breasts may have played an important role in lovemaking and your altered appearance will inevitably affect this. The ability to discuss these personal things with your partner and their willingness to respond to your needs rather than impose their own, will be important in restoring a sexual relationship. Many women find that this crisis brings them closer to their partners and that lovemaking is as good if not better than before.

Not all women have this experience. Some feel that the loss of a breast together with a scar line is deeply disfiguring. They can no longer look at themselves naked and cannot bear their sexual partners to do so either. They feel that losing a breast means losing part of their femininity. Unfortunately some men also have difficulty in coming to terms with the changed physical appearance of their wives and lovers.

If this is the case, it is important to seek help. Counsellors, clinical psychologists and psychotherapists have experience of working with women who feel distressed by their physical appearance. They can help you to gain confidence in yourself. Counsellors can also help couples to overcome the psychological barriers which become obstacles to lovemaking and intimacy.

Using a prosthesis and considering breast reconstruction

How you feel about wearing a breast-form and which kind suits you best will be something to experiment with after leaving hospital. Many women prefer to appear two-breasted but this won't be true for everyone. The important thing is for friends and relatives to respect your choice. This may mean they need to think through their own hang-ups about the female form and woman's sexuality.

More and more women are offered the choice of breast reconstruction after mastectomy. Some women take advantage of this, but others come to love their bodies as they are and feel no need for a constructed breast form. It's important not to let partners and friends or enthusiastic surgeons put pressure on you to make this choice. Womanhood and sexuality can never be reduced to the shape and symmetry of women's bodies. Whether you decide to have reconstruction surgery or not, must be *your* choice and no one else's.

Renewing your life

Gradually you will need to rebuild your confidence in your health. This may take courage and imagination. It can mean mapping out for yourself a whole-person health plan which takes account of your emotional and personal needs as well as your physical health. It probably take a little time to put together a plan which suits you and which doesn't overtax your strength. It may mean developing new skills and interests which you were unaware of before you had cancer. It may mean making new friends and relationships. The important thing is to find out what suits you and brings you most happiness and peace of mind.

> I've learnt to give myself permission to be a different kind of person really which is more like me. I'm not so workaholic and I'm not so uptight about so much. I just want to have more fun.

For many women, settling back to work and the friendships and acquaintances you had before you discovered cancer is a major adjustment. Most people will feel awkward and silent, not quite knowing what to say. You may find this irritating.

> I was confronted by a lady at work and she said: 'I'm very sorry that you've been ill,' meaning 'had cancer: the big "C"'. It was almost as if by now I would have this doom hanging over me because I'd had cancer and I was quite snappy with her. I said: 'I don't want people thinking I'm ill, I've *had* cancer but I don't have it now.'

You may find it useful to work out two or three responses if you find it a strain to deal with others' embarrassment or curiosity. You may find this helps you to avoid getting tense and irritated, for example:

> Actually I have had cancer and I'd rather everyone knew and not pretend that I haven't.

> I know you're trying to help but I'd prefer not to discuss it.

Living with cancer means coming to terms with the possibility of cancer spread and learning to put that fear in its place. Many women find that, to begin with, every ache and pain is suspected as evidence of spread and this causes great anxiety. It's only as time passes that the fear recedes. Each woman will find her own way of dealing with the fear of recurrence. Most recognize that coming to terms with this possibility is a major part of living with breast cancer.

> Coming to terms with cancer seems to require a major readjustment of attitudes and feelings. Even when there has been no recurrence, the frequent check-ups, in prospect for several years are bound to remind you that it *is* a strange disease which can keep a stubborn hold. You come to terms with it so that for most of the time you're no more aware of cancer than of having crooked teeth or flat feet; but I think to face it cheerfully you must not lose sight of the fact that we are *all* dying, and that since death is inevitable there is no point in worrying whether it will come tomorrow under a bus or in a few years' time in a hospice, or many years hence in a geriatric ward. You must get on with living, and life is really so full of good things.

It's important for all of us, whether we have cancer or not, to face up to the fear and the mythology surrounding this disease. Those of us who are cancer-free owe it to those who are not to be properly informed and worked-out about the meaning of cancer in our lives and in society as a whole.

Local recurrence and secondary spread

Roughly half the women who have breast cancer will have some form of recurrence of cancer. (These numbers are likely to decrease as cancers are treated earlier.) Recurrence can take two forms. Cancer can return in the breast tissue itself or it can form a secondary cancer in another part of the body. A minority of women will develop a second primary cancer in one of their breasts. Some cancers re-emerge twenty of thirty years after they are first found and many women with secondary spread will reach the end of their lives without any evidence of cancer symptoms.

Local recurrence A local recurrence of cancer in the breast is a setback but not necessarily more serious than the first discovery of cancer. Local recurrence does not necessarily mean that cancer has spread elsewhere. For this reason it is often treated in the same way as a primary cancer (see Chapters 12 to 16).

A second primary cancer A few women will get a second primary cancer either in the same breast or the other breast. This will also be treated as a primary cancer.

Secondary spread to other parts of the body Secondaries may develop in a number of areas in the body, for example in the spine or pelvis, in the lungs and in the liver. Cancer is an unpredictable disease which means that although the outlook may not be good for some women, this is not true for all women. Treatment will aim to control the symptoms for as long as possible. In some cases this will be for many years.

> I had a mastectomy 25 years ago and about eight years ago
> I developed secondaries in the spine and the pelvis. I was
> put on tamoxifen by my consultant. I was worried to begin
> with because I got more pain with the tamoxifen than before
> but that settled down and I've had no problems since. I'm
> determined not to let it beat me.

The treatment used as follow-up treatments for primary breast cancer are also used later if secondaries develop. The treatment to be used partly depends on where the secondary cancer is. It also depends on the degree of hormone sensitivity in the cancer. Radiotherapy, chemotherapy and tamoxifen can ease pain in secondary growths and in some cases shrink the cancer considerably. In hormone-sensitive cancers other hormone-related drugs can be used if tamoxifen or removal/irradiation of the ovaries become ineffective in containing the cancer. Progestogen (Provera and Farlutal) is a progesterone-like drug which can relieve pain and improve the quality of life in women with advanced disease. (Possible side-effects include weight changes, loss of periods, fine hand tremors and sweating.)

An alternative is to use drugs to influence hormonal activity in the adrenal glands situated near the kidneys. Orimeten, for example, can suppress the activity of oestrogen in body tissue in postmenopausal women. Secondary cancers can shrink and even disappear and pain can be relieved. The problem with these drugs (commonly called 'steroids') is that they affect other hormone activity as well which can eventually disrupt the body's different systems leading to altered fluid balance, replacement of muscles and skin with fat and an inability to deal with stress. While every effort is made to monitor any side-effects and replace hormones which have been suppressed, most people can expect some changes in the long term. If your consultant suggests steroids, it's advisable to ask about any side-effects before agreeing to treatment.

Traditional and complementary medicine will offer treatments which stimulate your body's healing capacity using the powers of the mind in visualization, meditation and hypnosis as well as diet, herbal drugs, acupuncture, massage, homoeopathic remedies and healing. You may prefer to choose these instead of or in combination with modern treatments.

Having secondary cancer is a worrying time for any woman. Renewed uncertainty can lead to distress and anxiety. An important thing to remember is that you are not alone. There are thousands of women in your situation, many of whom are continuing to live their lives to the full.

> Cancer seems always to have been part of my life. When I was 13 my mother had a mastectomy, radiotherapy and a lot of pain. She died three years later in 1937 at the age of 56. I first discovered that I had primary breast cancer in 1969. After surgery (a lumpectomy) and radiotherapy I was told I was 'clear'. After another 12 years however, inoperable (terminal) secondary cancers were found in my lymph glands, lung, etc. I was given a few months to live — a maximum of two years. That was nearly four years ago.
>
> Kit Mouat, *Spare Rib*, March, 1986

In that time Kit Mouat founded and helped to build Cancer Contact (three self-help groups for cancer patients) and she'd written a book (see Further reading). With help and support you, too, can discover new strengths in yourself to restore your courage and to renew your life at this difficult time.

Further reading

Sarah Boston and Jill Louw, *Disorderly Breasts* (Camden Press, 1987).

Penny Brohn, *Gentle Giants* (Century Paperbacks, 1987).

Jenny Bryan and Joanna Lyall, *Living with Cancer: What it is; where to get help; practical advice; forms of treatment* (Penguin Books, 1987).

Rachael Clyne, *Coping with Cancer: Making sense of it all* (Thorsons, 1986).

Ian Gawler, *You Can Conquer Cancer: The self-help guide to the way back to health* (Thorsons, 1986).

Brenda Kidman, *A Gentle Way with Cancer* (Century Paperbacks, 1983).

Rose Kushner, *Breast Cancer: A personal history and investigative report* (Harcourt Brace Jovanovich, 1976).

Audre Lorde, *The Cancer Journals* (Sheba Feminist Publications, 1985).

Kit Mouat, *Fighting for Our Lives: An introduction to living with cancer* (Heretic Books, 1984).

Nicholas Tarrier, *Living with Breast Cancer and Mastectomy* (Manchester University Press, 1987).

Betty Westgate, *Coping with Cancer* (The Breast Care and Mastectomy Association, 1987).

CHAPTER TWENTY
Living...and dying of breast cancer

For some women, the time may come when no further treatment can hope to cure breast cancer, or halt the spread of the disease. Instead treatment aims to ease any symptoms of pain and discomfort and increase the life span in the short term. For many women this situation may last years rather than months but for some women, the end of their lives may be very near.

In a society which hides from death and dying, preparing for death can be a distressing and sometimes frightening prospect. Living through these last months and coming to terms with dying means different things to different women. It may mean taking leave of friends and loved ones or settling your affairs. For some, it means renewing a faith in religion or finding a new source of knowledge and wisdom about your life. For many it will be a time of fear and worry.

This last chapter looks at some of the problems women face as patients and as carers in the last few months of life. It looks at ways of controlling pain and discomfort and outlines different avenues of personal support in living these last months as fully as possible.

Not all women will want to read this chapter yet all of us must face the possibility of dying at some time of our lives. Some of us will have begun that process already.

Those around you will want to comfort and support you, but they may need help in coming to terms with their own fears about death and dying in order to share with you your experiences, your fears and your hopes. Reading one of the books suggested at the end of this chapter may help you and those close to you to find a way of living positively with the possibility of dying. Hopefully this chapter will be helpful, too.

Relieving pain and discomfort

Most people associate dying of cancer with suffering. In fact relatively few people with cancer experience pain and these days, it can be successfully controlled. With breast cancer, pain is most likely when secondaries develop in the bones although some pain may be experienced if secondaries develop in the liver or the lungs. Some discomfort may be caused by side-effects of drugs (see comments on chemotherapy and hormone-related drugs in Chapter 16). With locally advanced cancer in the breast itself, a few women may develop ulceration which can also cause discomfort.

Pain management

You are the only person who will know whether or not you have pain and how severe it is. Tell the health professionals who care for you. Modern medicine is becoming far more skilled in the management of pain and can make your life pain-free and comfortable without loss of alertness. Non-steroid anti-inflammatory drugs and other hormone-related drugs (including tamoxifen and orimeten) may be offered for generalized pain. Drugs which block nerves to a particular part of the body can be given and radiotherapy can ease pain as well. Non-steroidal anti-inflammatory drugs can have some side-effects: the kidneys may be affected leading to water retention and the lining of the stomach can be affected. Vitamin E reduces kidney damage and aloe vera juice can reduce irritation in the lining of the stomach.

There are also effective ways of controlling pain using acupuncture, hypnosis, healing and relaxation therapies. Many women have found that these methods have enabled them to reduce their reliance on drugs and have improved their quality of life.

Physical discomfort

Locally advanced breast cancer is not always accompanied with secondary cancers elsewhere but this is usually the case. The breast can become inflamed and eventually produce an open wound (particularly if the cancer is near the surface of the breast) which may have an unpleasant smelling discharge. With proper care, the wound can remain clear and odourless and easily dressed. The Royal College of Nursing has produced a booklet for district nurses and others on the management of ulcerated breast cancer which gives detailed suggestions on the care and treatment of this condition. It can be distressing to develop an ulcerated area in the breast but remember that district nurses and home-care support teams can give you very effective help in controlling this condition, allowing you to live your life as normally as possible.

Treatments which aim to lengthen life

As well as helping with the management of pain, hormone-related drugs are used to lengthen life by weeks and sometimes months in cancers which are hormone-sensitive. In other cases chemotherapy may be suggested. There is increasing debate within the medical profession about the value of chemotherapy to prolong a woman's life when the side-effects of these toxic drugs undermine the quality of life in the remaining weeks or months (see page 144).

Avenues of support

You may need space apart from your family and friends to talk about your feelings about dying. You may need support in arranging your affairs. Perhaps you want to make a will or have strong feelings about where you want to die. You may also wish to give clear instructions about any treatment aimed at prolonging your life.

Through the work of the hospice movement and people like Elisabeth Kubler-Ross, there is now greater awareness of the need to support those who are facing death and to respect their wishes in whatever choices they make. Counsellors, social workers and psychotherapists can help you work through your feelings about dying. They can help you to resolve any nagging worries and regrets you may have and can act on your wishes, should you want any arrangements made.

Family members and other carers can also benefit from such support. Some of the worry and grief of losing a loved one can begin to be helped by a counsellor or therapist.

Your doctor or your nearest hospice will be able to put you in touch with someone who can help you and those close to you.

The role of hospices

A hospice is a place which provides special care for whom no cure is possible. Hospices have developed knowledge and experience in providing emotional and physical support for patients, including the effective management of pain. Their approach is based on respect for the wishes of each individual and they will, if you wish, combine modern and traditional or complementary remedies for pain.

Hospices can provide nursing care at home in a day-care unit as well as for in-patients. Unlike hospital, a hospice is a relaxed, hospitable place with pleasant rooms and varied menus. A hospice aims to provide support for the needs of each individual and those close to them. You may be invited to enter a hospice for a while so that any problems with pain or discomfort can be treated, or to ease the responsibility of those who care for you so that they can have a short rest. At home you will be supported by a home care team until such time as you wish to return. It will be your own wishes which are acted upon.

All workers in the hospice from doctors to cleaners have time to share with you. They are there to support you in the moments of grief *and* the moments of joy and laughter.

> What I'll always remember is the happiness and laughter in the hospice for Mum and me. I might feel low coming to the hospice but the moment I walked through the door, my spirits lightened.

Hospices are open to anyone who needs hospice care. Some hospices are run by the NHS and others are run by charitable donations and fund-raising. You are invited to give a donation to privately run hospices, if you can afford to, but no one is charged for hospice care. There are still far too few hospices in Britain which means resources are limited but it is worth contacting the hospice in your area. They will help you in any way they can.

A time for living and a time for dying

Coming to terms with the possibility of dying takes time. In our society death is seen as a private, individual event which each of us must face alone, and this can be very frightening. Elisabeth Kubler-Ross has pioneered work in understanding this process. She suggests that people go through different stages as they approach death beginning with denial that life will end. She suggests that people will express anger at their situation and try to bargain for extra time. Recognizing the loss of a future brings grief and depression and it is only gradually that acceptance of the situation allows the individual to begin to let go.

It's important that carers try to understand the nature of the crisis their friends and partners go through in coming to terms with dying. For those who don't believe in an afterlife or an all-loving God, other meanings can be found which provide a frame-work for living these months, days, moments in peace and har-mony, with ourselves as part of the wider cycles of life and death in nature, in the passing of the seasons and in the renewal of life outside the individual. We have few words to describe these things and each woman will find her own meaning in coming to terms with death.

Our choices are as real in these last months as at any other time. We may choose to spend the time quietly with those who are close to us. We may decide to refuse any further treatment.

> I have begun the process of dying. The chemotherapy is no longer working to control the cancer and there is very little that medical knowledge can do for me now. I have chosen, rather than to have salvage chemotherapy (which is what they call the stuff that barely works), to live my life as fully as possible, to live well and to die comfortably, in peace and calm, with friends and loved ones surrounding me. I feel extremely peaceful about my decisions. Occasional pain in the liver is the only discomfort I feel and, for that, I have pain medication.

There may be unfinished business which we need to complete before the time is right to 'let go'.

> I first met Wendy when she was quite ill. She had secon-daries in her spine which made walking difficult. Her lungs and her liver were also affected and she'd recently been told she had secondaries in her brain. This was causing some problems with her vision.
> Wendy had lived and worked in Zimbabwe for several years and so she decided to make a three-month visit to see friends and to see the country and the people she was deeply com-mitted to. We talked briefly about death and she thought that maybe she might die in Zimbabwe.

Wendy spent her three months in Zimbabwe. She was taken ill on the flight home to Britain and died shortly after in a London hospital. Women have many things to learn from each other. We can learn to find the courage and determination to live our lives to the full and we can share our fears and distress in times of crisis. With those who are dying and those who survive, we have a wealth of experience to share and understand.

Coming to terms with loss

Mourning the loss of a partner or friend will take time and may need the help of a bereavement counsellor or psychotherapist or the support of a cancer self-help group. It means thinking through the meaning of death and finding ways of honouring the person you loved. A funeral service may help to acknowledge this or a meeting of friends to share memories, photographs and music. Some people will want to make some symbolic act like planting a tree in memory of their loved one. Others may want to create a more general memorial, such as a trust fund. This time of grieving can provide the opportunity to work out in what ways the person you have lost lives on.

Further reading

Directory of Hospice Services, St Christopher's Hospice Information Service, 51 Lawrie Park Road, Sydenham, London SE26 6DZ.

Stephen Fulder, *How to Survive Medical Treatment: a holistic approach to the risks and side-effects of orthodox medicine* (Century Paperbacks, 1987).

Ian Gawler, *You Can Conquer Cancer: The self-help guide to the way back to health* (Thorsons, 1986).

Elisabeth Kubler-Ross, *On Death and Dying* (Collier Macmillan, 1973) gives a very positive approach to the subject.

Stephen Levine, *Who dies? An investigation of conscious living and conscious dying* (Gateway Books, 1988). This is a long book so probably the best way of using it is to dip into it and take what you find useful.

Denise Winn, *The Hospice Way* (Optima, 1987).

Useful addresses

Official bodies of modern medicine
British Medical Association, Tavistock Square, London WC1H 9JP. 01-387 4499.

Department of Health and Social Society, Alexander Fleming House, Elephant and Castle, London SE1 6BY. 01-404 5522.

Bodies giving general information
The British Holistic Medical Association, 179 Gloucester Place, London NW1 6DX. 01-262 5299.

The College of Health, 18 Victoria Park Square, Bethnal Green, London E2 9PF. 01-980 6263.

The Institute of Complementary Medicine, 21 Portland Place, London W1N 3AF. 01-636 9543.

The Women's Health and Reproductive Rights Information Centre, 52-54, Featherstone St, London EC1. 01-251 6332/6580.

Bodies concerned with patient's rights
Association of Community Health Councils, 30 Drayton Park, London N5 1PB. 01-609 8405.

National Consumer Council, Grosvenor Gardens, London SW1. 01-730 3469.

Patients' Association, Room 33, 18 Charing Cross Rd, London WC2H 0HR. 01-240 0671.

Professional bodies and registers of practitioners in traditional and complementary medicine
Anthroposophical Medical Association, The Old Forge, Bell End, Belbroughton, Stourbridge DY9 9UD. 0562 730362 and 01-723 4400/8219.

The Association of Therapeutic Healers, 95 Constantine Rd, London NW3 2LP. 01-485 7656, 240 0176, 267 4674.

Bach Flower Remedies Ltd, Dr Edward Bach Centre, Mount Vernon, Sotwell, Wallingford, Oxon OX10 0PZ. 0491 39489.

British Acupuncture Association and Register, 34 Alderney St, London SW1V 4EU. 01-834 1012/3353.

British Association of Art Therapists, 13c Northwood Rd, London N6 5TL.

The British Homoeopathic Association, 27a Devonshire Rd, London W1N 1RJ. 01-935 2163.

British Medical Acupuncture Society, Newton House, Newton Lane, Lower Whitley, Warrington, Cheshire WA4 4JA. 092 573727.

The British Naturopathic and Osteopathic Association, 6 Netherall Gardens, London NW3 5RR. 01-435 8728.

British Society for Music Therapy, 69 Avondale Avenue, East Barnet, Herts EN4 8NB. 01-368 8879.

British Tai Chi Ch'uan Association, 7 Upper Wimpole St, London W1M 7TD. 01-935 8444.

The College of Dietary Therapy, Hillsborough House, Ashley, Tiverton, Devon EX16 5PA. 0884 255879.

Community Health Foundation, 188 Old St, London EC1V 9BP. 01-251 4076. (Traditional Japanese and Chinese medicine).

Federation of Spiritual Healers, Old Manor Farm Studio, Church St, Sudbury-on-Thames, Middx TW16 6RG. 0932 783164/5.

The General Council and Register of Consultant Herbalists Ltd, Marlborough House, Swanpool, Falmouth, Cornwall TR11 4HW. 0326 317321.

Homoeopathic Development Foundation, Suite 1, 19a Cavendish Square, London W1M 9AD. 01-629 320415.

The Incorporated Society of Registered Naturopaths, 328 Harrogate Rd, Moortown, Leeds LS17 6PE. 0532 685992.

The Institute of Allergy Therapists, Ffynnonwen, Llangwyryfon, Aberystwyth, Dyfed SY23 4EY. 09747 376.

Institute of Psychosynthesis, 1 Cambridge Gate, Regent's Park, London NW1 4JN. 01-486 2588.

Matthew Manning Centre, 39 Abbeygate St, Bury St Edmunds, Suffolk IP33 1LW. 0284 69502/752364.

National Association of Hypnotists and Psychotherapists, Aberystwyth, Dyfed SY23 4EY. 09747 376.

National Council and Register of Iridology, 80 Portland Rd, Bournemouth, Dorset BH9 1NQ. 0202 529793.

The National Institute of Medical Herbalists, 41 Hatherley Rd, Winchester, Hants SO22 6RR. 0962 68776.

The Osteopathic and Naturopathic Guild Ltd, Marlborough House, Swanpool, Falmouth, Cornwall TR11 4HW. 0326 317321.

Register of Traditional Chinese Herbal Medicine, 7a Stanhope Rd, London N6. 01-348 2470.

Register of Traditional Chinese Medicine, 19 Trinity Rd, London N2 8JJ. 01-883 8432.

Society of Homoeopaths, 11a Bampton St, Tiverton, Devon EX16 6HH. 0884 3091.

Society of Teachers of the Alexander Technique, 10 London House, 266 Fulham Rd, London SW10 9EL. 01-351 0828.

Traditional Acupuncture Association, 11 Grange Park, Stratford-upon-Avon, CV7 6XH. 0789 298798.

Organizations which test for vitamin and mineral deficiency and give advice on dietary supplements

Healthlink Ltd, Hillsborough House, Ashley, Tiverton, Devon EX16 5PA. 0884 252027.

G R Lane Healthcrafts Ltd, 203-205 Sissons Rd, Gloucester GL1 3QB. 0452 24012.

Nature's Best, 1 Lamberts Rd, Tunbridge Wells, Kent TN2 3EQ. 0892 34143.

Nature's Own Ltd, West Malvern Rd, West Malvern, Worcs WR14 4BB. 06845 63465.

Nutricare Ltd (Gerrard House), 736 Christchurch Rd, Bournemouth, Hants. 0202 35352.

NHS homoeopathic hospitals

Bristol Homoeopathic Hospital, Cotham Rd, Cotham, Bristol BS6 6JU.

The Glasgow Homoeopathic Hospital, 1000 Great Western Rd, Glasgow G12 0RN.

Liverpool Clinic, Mossley Hill Hospital, Park Avenue, Liverpool, L18 8BU.

The Royal London Homoeopathic Hospital, Great Ormond St, London WC1N 3HR. 01-837 3091.

Tunbridge Wells Homoeopathic Hospital, Church Rd, Tunbridge Wells, Kent.

Organizations giving specialist information about cancer and treatments

BACUP (British Association of Cancer United Patients and their Families and Friends, 121/123 Charterhouse St, London EC1M 6AA. 01-608 1661 (see below).

CancerLink, 46 Pentonville Rd, London N1 9HF. 01-833 2451 (see below).

The Jeannie Campbell Appeal, 29 St Luke's Avenue, Ramsgate, Kent, CT11 7J2. 0843 596732/593193.

New Approaches to Cancer, c/o the Seekers Trusts, Addington Park, Maidstone, Kent, ME19 5BL. 0732 848336.

Women's Cancer Control Campaign, 1 South Audley Street, London W1Y 5DQ. 01-499 7532.

Cancer help centres for complementary treatments for cancer

Bournemouth Centre of Complementary Medicine, 26 Sea Rd, Boscombe, Bournemouth, Dorset BH5 1DF. 0202 36354.

Bristol Cancer Help Centre, Grove House, Cornwallis Grove, Bristol BS8 4PG. 0272 743216.

The Gentle Approach to Cancer Association, c/o 104 Millans Court, Ambleside, Cumbria LA22 9BN. 05394 32627, 09662 3337, 07687 73267.

Park Attwood Centre, Trimbley, Bewdley, Worcs. DY12 1RE. 02997 444.

Wessex Cancer Help Centres, 8 South St, Chichester, West Sussex PO19 1EH. 0243 778516.

New Approaches to Cancer holds a list of centres and practitioners throughout the British Isles (see above).

Support organizations

BACUP provides advice and emotional support for cancer patients and their families.

The Breast Care and Mastectomy Association, 26 Harrison St, Off Gray's Inn Road, Kings Cross, London WC1H 8JG. 01-837 0908. It gives support and information to any woman who contacts them. It trains volunteer visitors who will go and talk to women who have breast cancer or who have had treatment for the disease and it co-ordinates a national network of self-help groups.

Cancerlink also co-ordinates a national network of cancer support and self-help groups and helps new groups who are in the process of setting up.

Cancer — You Are Not Alone (CYANA), 31 Church Rd, Manor Park, London E12 6AD. 01-553 5366 and 553 0333.

Information about hospices and terminal care

Hospice Information, St Christopher's Hospice, 51/59 Lawrie Park, Sydenham, London SE26 6DZ. 01-778 9252.

Macmillan Nurses, c/o The National Society for Cancer Relief, Anchor House, 15-19 Britten St, London SW3 3TY. 01-351 7811.

List of technical and unusual words

This is a list of all the technical or unusual words used in this book. Some additional technical terms are also included which you may hear doctors use during investigation of a breast problem.

Abscess a painful, boil-like infection beneath the skin.

Acupressure a part of Chinese medicine which uses finger and hand pressure at different points in the body. Acupressure is used in China and elsewhere to relieve pain and to treat disease.

Acupuncture a part of Chinese medicine which uses fine needles to puncture the skin at different points in the body. Acupuncture is used in China and elsewhere to relieve pain and to treat disease.

Adenoma non-cancerous growth in glandular body tissue.

Adjuvant means back-up or additional. It is used when talking about further treatments for cancer, e.g. chemotherapy.

Alexander Technique complementary therapy which aims to increase well-being through exercise to improve posture and movement.

Alopecia loss of hair on the body, particularly the head.

Amenorrhea the absence of periods.

Amygdalin an extract from fruit pips and kernels thought by some doctors to help in the treatment of cancer.

Anthroposophy an alternative therapy based on the philosophy of Rudolf Steiner.

Antibody part of the immune system's ability to protect the body from disease.

Antigen signals displayed by cells.

Anti-oxidant a substance which protects the body from the harmful effects of oxidation (natural anti-oxidants include vitamin E, beta-carotene and selenium)

Areola the circular area of dark skin surrounding the nipple.

Arteries channels which carry the blood away from the heart (a part of the cadio-vascular system).

Aspiration a means of withdrawing fluid from body tissue using a needle attached to a syringe.

Axilla armpit.
Ayurveda traditional Hindu medicine practised widely in India.

Bach flower remedies flower essences used to treat emotional states.
Bacteria tiny organisms found in plants and animals. They range from harmless to disease-producing and some are very dangerous.
Benign tumour non-cancerous growth which does not invade other tissue or travel to other sites in the body.
Biopsy removal of a small amount of body tissue which is then studied carefully in a laboratory.

Capilliary very small blood vessels which service body tissue.
Carcinogen any substance which can bring about cancerous changes in the cells of humans or animals.
Carcinoma a cancerous growth of epithelial cells which line the body's external and internal surfaces like the skin, large intestine, lungs, stomach, cervix and breast (ducts and channels). Carcinomas invade surrounding tissue and tend to travel through the body to other sites where they form new growths.
Carcinoma in situ a cancerous growth which does not invade surrounding tissue or travel to new sites. It occurs in the milk lobules.
Cardio-vascular system the network of blood vessels (including veins, arteries and capilliaries) together with the heart which channels blood throughout the body.
Cell differentiation the process by which cells of a common origin take on different functions and characteristics. Well differentiated cells behave normally while poorly differentiated cells have lost a number of functions and characteristics like their timer mechanism for cell reproduction.
Chemotherapy treatment by one or more drugs which are capable of destroying cancer cells and other quickly reproducing cells.
Chronic persisting or long lasting.
Circumscribed carcinoma in a well-defined cancer with a capsule-like outer layer.
Clinical trials carefully organized tests which aim to measure the effectiveness of particular treatments for a disease.
Colostrum rich milky fluid which the breast produces in the first few days of childbirth.
Consultant senior doctor specializing in a particular area of medicine.
Cortisone cream hormonal cream. (It can be used to treat skin affected by radiotherapy.)
Cyst a sac filled with fluid usually soft to the touch, but sometimes quite hard and round.
Cystosarcoma phyllodes similar to a fibroadenoma but tends to produce a harder lump which sometimes grows quite large.
Cytology the study of cells.
Cytoplasm the substance which forms the main part of a cell.

Cytotoxic drugs drugs used to damage and destroy cancer cells.

Differentiation see cell differentiation
Diuretic drug which helps fluid retention by increasing the volume of urine.
DNA genetic blueprint in the nucleus (DNA stands for deoxyribonucleic acid).
Drill and tru-cut biopsy biopsy using a wide bore needle attached to a syringe.
Duct a tube-like channel which can carry fluid — there are milk ducts in the breasts.
Duct ectasia enlarging and eventually hardening of a diseased duct accompanied by discharge from the nipple.
Dysplasia abnormal tissue growth. Generally used to describe non-cancerous cell changes.

Endocrine system the system of hormones circulating in the body.
Enema a solution given through the anus to open and clear out the bowels.
Environment all the different things in our lives which effect us socially, physically and personally, e.g. pollution, diet, housing, income, weather.
Enzyme a protein produced in a cell which affects cell function and behaviour.
Epithelium sheet of cells forming the lining of tubes, cavities and surfaces in the body. Most cancers occur in the epithelial cells.
Excision removal of body tissue using surgery.

Fat necrosis the death of fat cells which can form a lump in the breast.
Fibroadenoma a non-cancerous growth of fibrous and glandular tissue. Fibroadenosis is a more generalized spread of this condition. A lactational adenoma is a fibroadenoma which develops during pregnancy.
Fibrocystic disease a non-cancerous condition involving cysts and fibrous tissue.
Fibrous tissue body tissue consisting of fibres, sometimes increased as a response to disease.
Fibrosis thickening of lumpiness in fibrous tissue.
Free radicals substances present in food which can damage DNA.
Frozen section a biopsy performed and studied while a patient is under a general anaesthetic. The tissue sample is rapidly frozen to enable speedy investigation.

Gene a section of DNA which contains the information necessary for an inherited characteristic, e.g. eye colour.
Gentian violet purple antiseptic dye painted on to skin.
Glands structures in the body which produce and send out hormones to different parts of the body, e.g. the ovaries.

Histology the study of body tissue.

Homoeopathy a system of medicine based on the principles of 'like cures like' using methods of dilution and shaking with the aim of producing safe remedies of different strengths for the treatment of disease.

Hormone chemical message which triggers changes in cell behaviour.

Hormone replacement therapy (HRT) hormonal treatment used to replace levels of oestrogen, used during and after the menopause.

Hospice a place which provides special care for those who are dying.

Hydrotherapy therapy using water, e.g. sprays, bathing, swimming.

Hyperplasia increased cell production.

Hysterectomy surgical removal of the womb.

Immune system the body's system for self-healing and protection from disease.

Immunotherapy treatment which aims to increase the efficiency of the immune system.

Implant (breast) an artificial breast-form usually made of silicon which is placed beneath the skin or chest muscle after a mastectomy or in a separate operation.

Inflammatory breast cancer painful but rare cancer providing generalized inflammation in the breast.

In situ refers to non-invasive cancers. (Latin for inplace).

Intraductal cancer non-invasive cancer which occurs in the milk ducts.

Intraductal papilloma see *Papilloma*

Invasive cancer cancer which spreads into surrounding tissue.

Ionizing radiation rays of very small particles capable of damaging the genetic structure of fast growing cells, e.g. X-rays.

Iscador an extract of mistletoe which is thought to increase the effectiveness of the immune system.

Keloid lumpy scar tissue.

Lactation milk production for breast feeding in mammals.

Lactational adenoma see *Fibroadenoma*.

Leukemia a cancer of the white cells in the blood supply.

Ligament a band of fibrous tissue joining or binding the body structure together. Cooper's ligaments hold the breast against the chest wall.

Lipoma a non-cancerous growth of fatty tissue.

Lobe a rounded division of an organ. A lobule is a small lobe.

Lobular carcinoma in situ a non-invasive cancer of the lobules.

Lumpectomy the surgical removal of a breast lump.

Lymph a fluid flowing through body tissue similar to blood.

Lymph nodes a small mass of tissue where lymph is cleared and lymphocytes are found in large numbers.

Lymphatic system the network of channels which carry lymph around the body.

Lymphocytes cells which form an important part of the body's immune response.

Lymphoedema accumulation of lymph causing swelling. Can occur as a result of damage or removal of the lymph nodes.

Macrophages specialized cells which play an important part in the body's immune system.

Malignant growth a cancerous growth.

Mammals all animals which breastfeed their young.

Mammary glands specialized milk-producing glands in all mammals.

Mammogram breast X-ray.

Mammography science of breast examination by X-ray.

Mastalgia breast pain.

Mastectomy surgical removal of the breast.

Mastitis a general term used to describe inflammation of the breast. Often used more loosely to cover a number of breast conditions. Plasma cell or periductal mastitis is caused by chemical changes in breast tissue, not by infection.

Medullary breast cancer a cancer which forms a well-defined lump with a capsule-like outer layer.

Megadose very large dose.

Menopause the time, usually between 45 and 55, when a woman stops having periods. This marks the end of a woman's reproductive life.

Menstruation monthly periods.

Metaplasia changes in cell structure which may lead to disease.

Metastasis the spread of cells from a primary cancer to form a secondary cancer site in the body. The plural is metastases.

Micro-metastasis tiny groups of cancerous cells which have spread from a primary cancer.

Mitosis the process of cell division.

Modified radical mastectomy surgical removal of the breast, together with the lymph nodes.

Mucinous breast cancer a type of cancer in which the cancerous cells produce a mucus-like substance.

Naturopathy a system of therapy using only 'natural' treatment and remedies.

Necrosis death of tissue.

Neoplasia new and unnecessary cell growth.

Neoplasm new tumour. Cancers are sometimes referred to as neoplasms.

Non-invasive cancer cancer which does not spread.

Nucleus that part of the cell in plants and animals which contains the genetic information for cell growth and reproduction.

Nutrients food substances like proteins, fats and carbohydrates. These can be microscopic in cell nutrients.

Oedema swelling caused by fluid build-up in body tissue.

Oestrogen hormone produced by the ovaries which plays an important role in a woman's reproductive cycle.

Oncogenes genes thought to be responsible for triggering the development of some cancers.

Oncologist a cancer specialist who may be responsible for an overall plan of treatment for cancer.

Oncology the study and practice of treatments for cancer.

Oopherectomy surgical removal of the ovaries.

Osteoporosis a condition where the bones become brittle and painful due to mineral deficiency.

Oxytocin a hormone which triggers milk production in breastfeeding.

Paget's disease an unusual form of cancer producing a skin rash in the nipple similar to eczema.

Palpation examination using the hand to feel — a palpable lump is one you can feel.

Papilliary breast cancer a cancer which grows in a similar way to a intraductal papilloma.

Papilloma a small non-cancerous growth like a wart. An intraductal papilloma growing in a milk duct of the breast.

Partial mastectomy removal of a wedge-like portion of breast tissue.

Pathology the biological study of disease and its causes.

Pectoral muscle the chest muscles which lie immediately behind the breast.

Peri-operatively during or immediately after an operation.

Pituitary gland a gland situated within the skull which plays an important role in the production of different hormones.

Placenta the life-chord linking the unborn baby to the womb of a pregnant woman. The placenta is responsible for the development and well-being of the foetus up to birth.

Postmenopausal after the change of life when periods cease.

Post-operatively after surgery.

Precancerous cells abnormal cells which may develop into cancer, but not always.

Premenstrual before a period.

Premenopausal before the change of life (when periods cease).

Pre-operatively before surgery.

Primary cancer a first cancerous tumour from which secondaries may spread.

Progesterone a hormone produced by the ovaries which plays an important role in women's reproductive lives.

Prognosis working out the likely course of events of a disease.

Prolactin a hormone which controls the production of milk in a woman who is breastfeeding.

Prosthesis an artificial limb or substitute for a part of the body.

Puberty the beginning of sexual maturity.

Pyrodoxine another name of vitamin B_6.

Quadrectomy see *Partial mastectomy.*

Radiation rays of very small particles, e.g. sun light, heat, X-rays.

Radical or classical mastectomy the surgical removal of the breast, the underlying chest muscles and the axillary lymph nodes. A *super-radical mastectomy* removes the internal chain of lymph nodes lying beneath the breast bone, as well. *Modified mastectomy* removes only the breast tissue and lymph nodes in th armpit.

Radiotherapy a treatment using ionizing radiation with the aim of destroying cancer cells.

Radium a substance which gives off ionizing radiation.

Registrar a hospital doctor who is responsible to a consultant.

Remission a period of good health after a disease has developed. This may happen naturally or may be due to a particular treatment.

Sarcoma cancers which form in connective tissue like muscle, fat, bone or cartilage.

Sclerosing adenosis a non-cancerous breast condition caused by new glandular growth which has become hardened or 'sclerosed'.

Secondaries cancers which develop from cells spread from a primary tumour.

Segmentectomy see partial mastectomy.

Silicon implant artificial material inserted by surgery into the breast to make it larger.

Simulator X-ray machine used to monitor the effects of radiotherapy on the breast and surrounding tissue.

Simple mastectomy breast removal where the underlying chest muscles and the lymph nodes are left intact.

Sinuses small collecting reservoirs existing in different parts of the body. During breastfeeding milk collects in sinuses in the breast.

Steroid drugs hormonal drugs.

Subcutaneous under the skin.

Subcutaneous mastectomy removal of underlying breast tissue leaving the skin and nipple intact.

Systemic relating to the whole system or whole body.

T'ai Chi Chuan traditional Chinese exercise.

Tissue a general term for groups of cells in the body usually with a particular function, e.g. the breast or the liver.

Therapy another word for treatment and usually covers every type of treatment or remedy.

Toxic poisonous.

Tru-cut biopsy see drill biopsy.

Tubular breast cancer cancer in which the cells form a tube-like pattern.

Ulceration the development of an ulcer in the body.

Ultrasound a means of scanning body tissue and organs using sound waves.

Veins blood vessels which return blood from body tissue and lungs to the heart.

Virus an infectious agent carrying disease.

Visualization a therapy where a patient pictures the healing process within their bodies. Used in many different situations including cancer therapy.

Vitamins food factors, essential to the well-being of humans, present in many natural foods.

Index